Diet and Exercise
MOTIVATIONS
Coloring Book

30 Motivational Words Coloring Designs

I've Got This Journals

© 2016 by I've Got This Journals
© 2016 Cover design and editing by Jen Schaefer

All rights reserved. No part of this publication may be reproduced, distributed, or transmitted in any form or by any means, including photocopying, recording, or other electronic or mechanical methods, without the prior written permission of the publisher, except in the case of brief quotations embodied in critical reviews and certain other noncommercial uses permitted by copyright law.

ISBN-13: 978-1537742786
ISBN-10: 1537742787

The Diet and Exercise Motivations Coloring Book is a great addition to use along with the Diet and Exercise Journals by *I've Got This* Journals, which are available in 8 cover designs all with the same great interior.

The Diet and Exercise Motivations Coloring Book provides a fun outlet to color (instead of unhealthy snacking) and focus on the encouraging word(s) found on each coloring page. It's sized a bit larger than the Journals to give you plenty of coloring fun on each design. Now you can color to relax as well as focus on your healthy diet and exercise plan that you're tracking in your journal. Each of the 30 motivational words coloring designs are on one side only- and each coloring design also has extra space beneath so you can "free style" notes.

Let us know how you're enjoying the **Diet and Exercise Motivations Coloring Book** by *I've Got This* Journals - we look forward to hearing from you! Your feedback is appreciated via reviews and/or email: journals@ivegotthisjournals.com

Find out more about I've Got This Journals' paperback journals:
I've Got This Diet and Exercise Journals are designed for everyone who wants to increase their success rate in losing weight by keeping a food journal. *I've Got This* Journals give you a place to formalize and record your plan - and much more.

Change Is Good

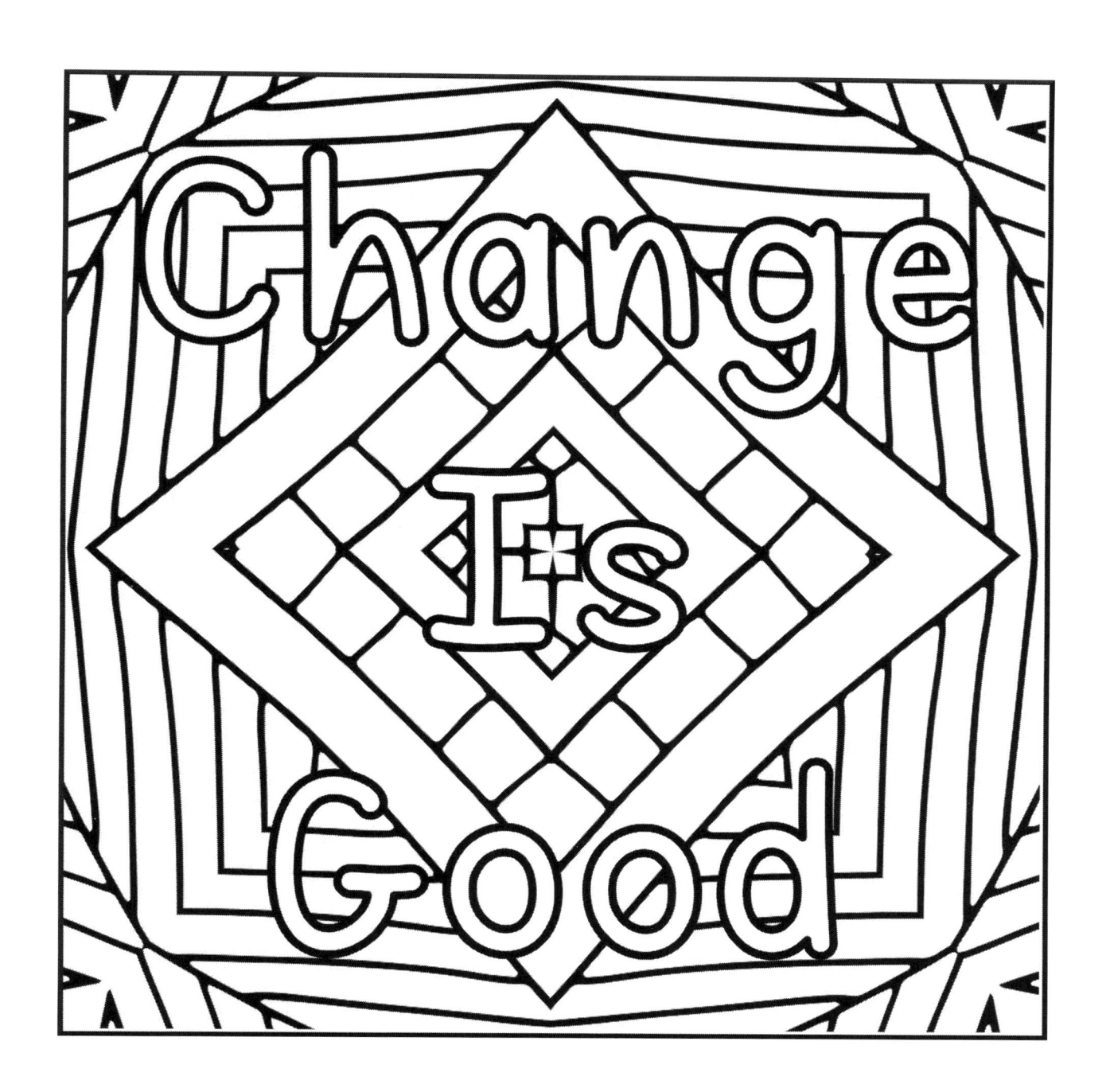

I Can Do This

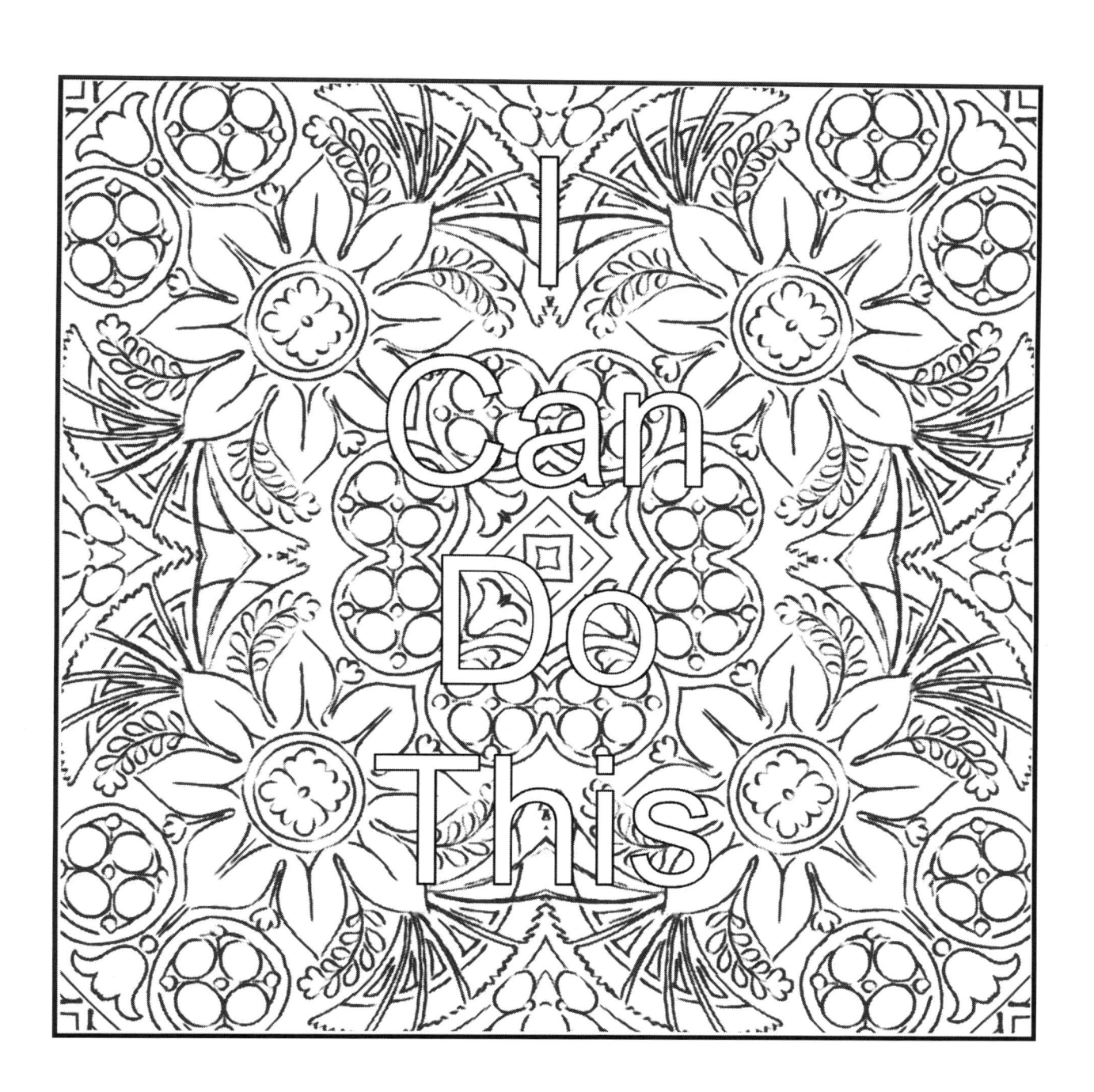

Never Give Up

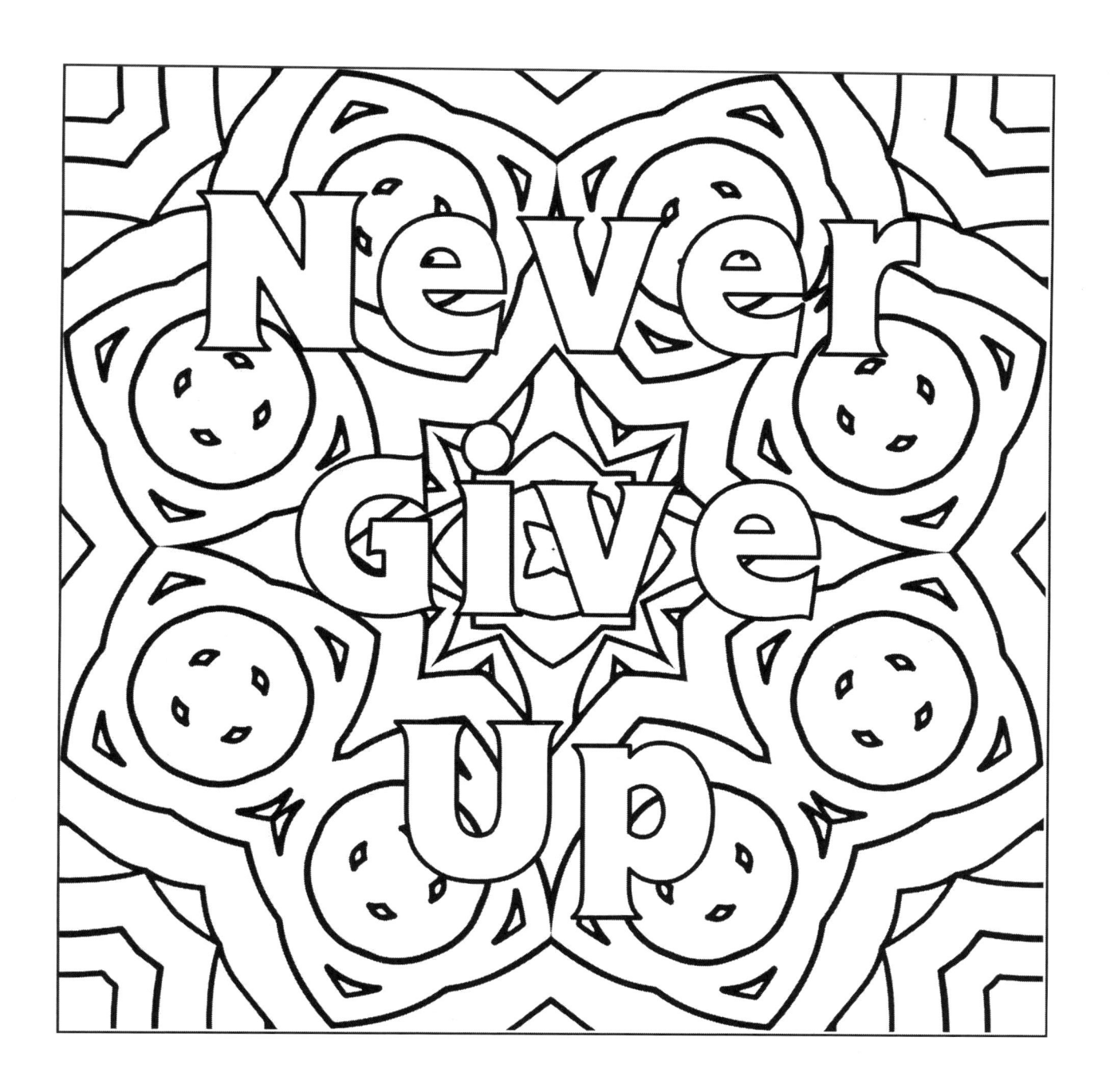

Set your Goals

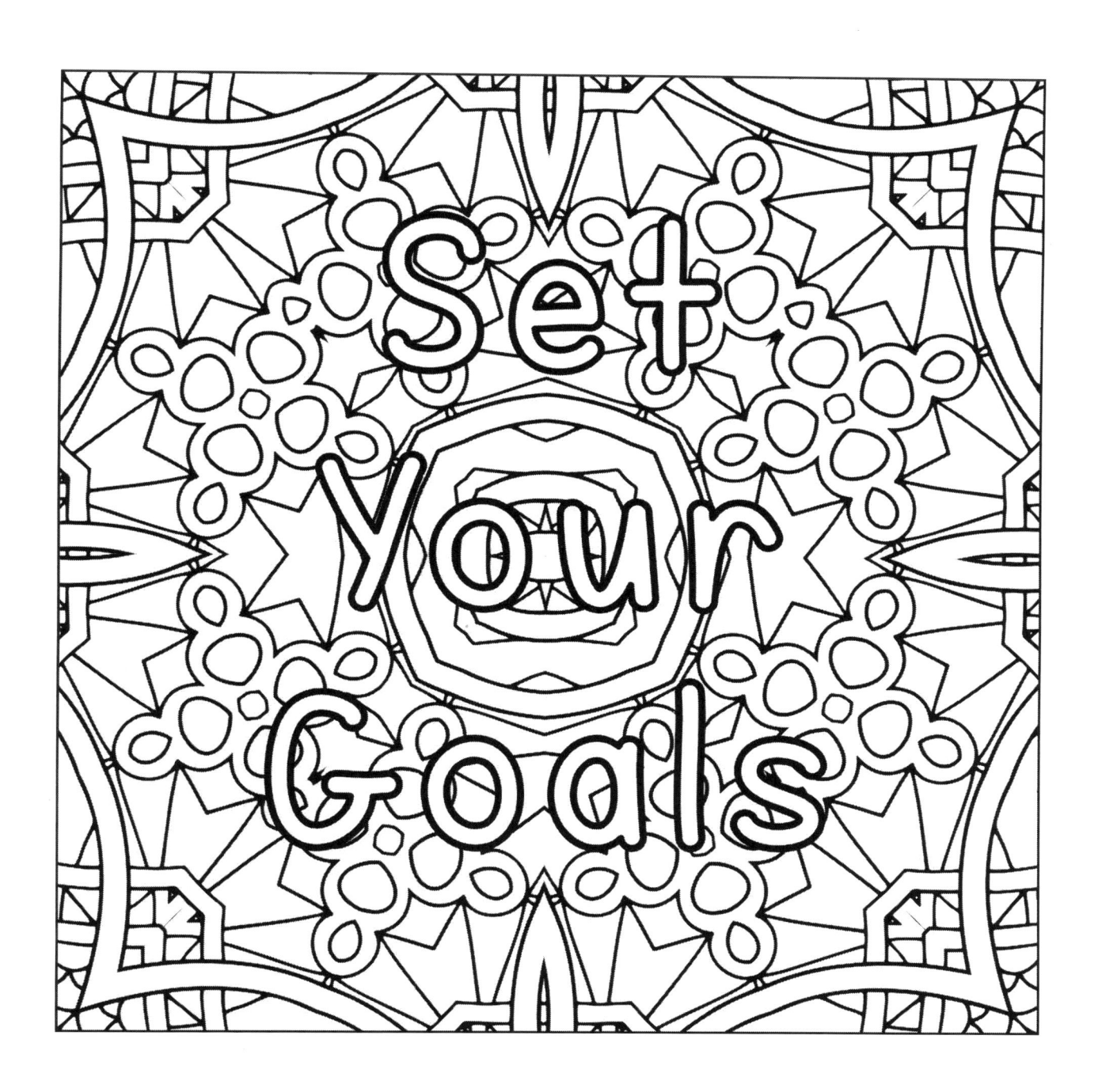

Make Your Own Path

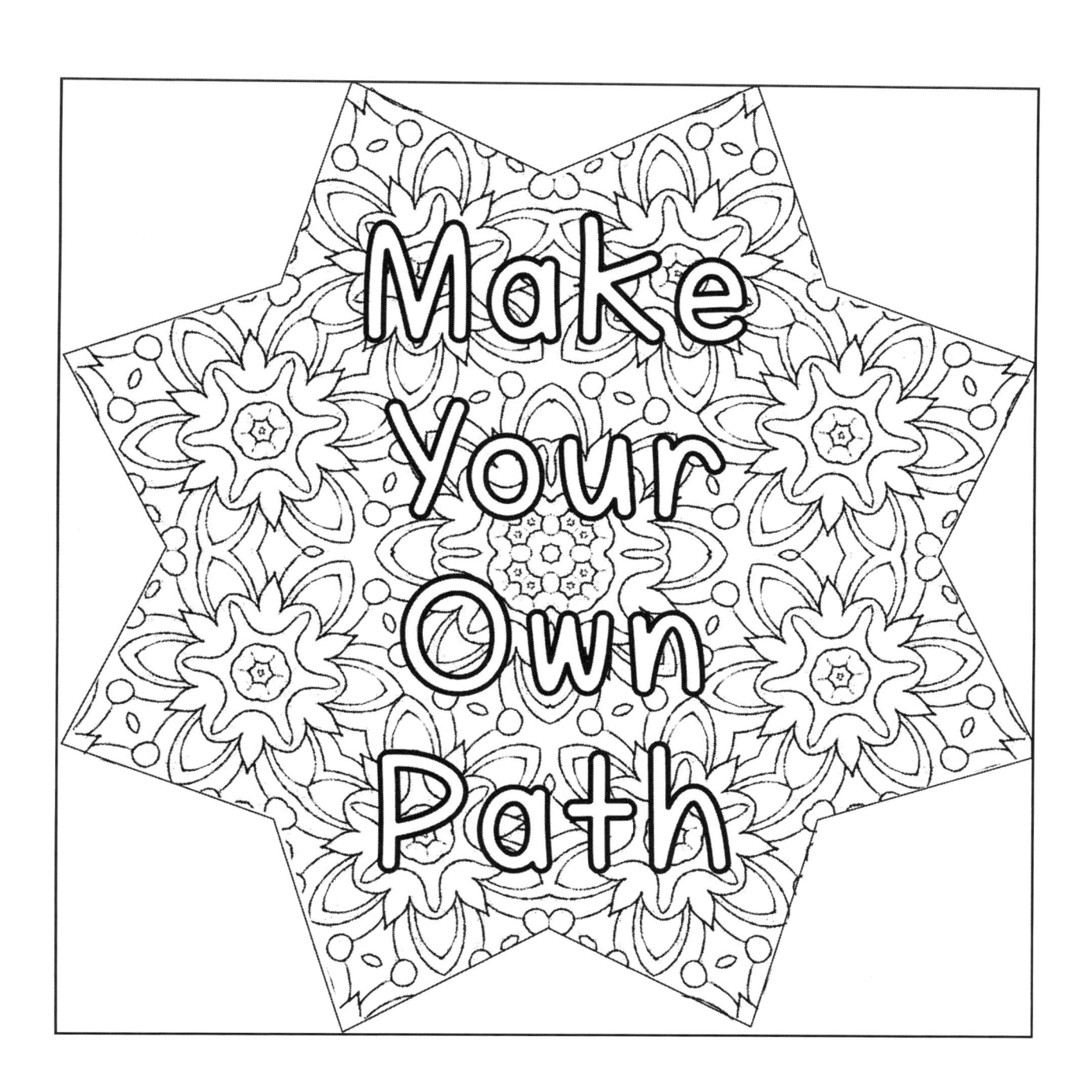

Nourish Your Soul

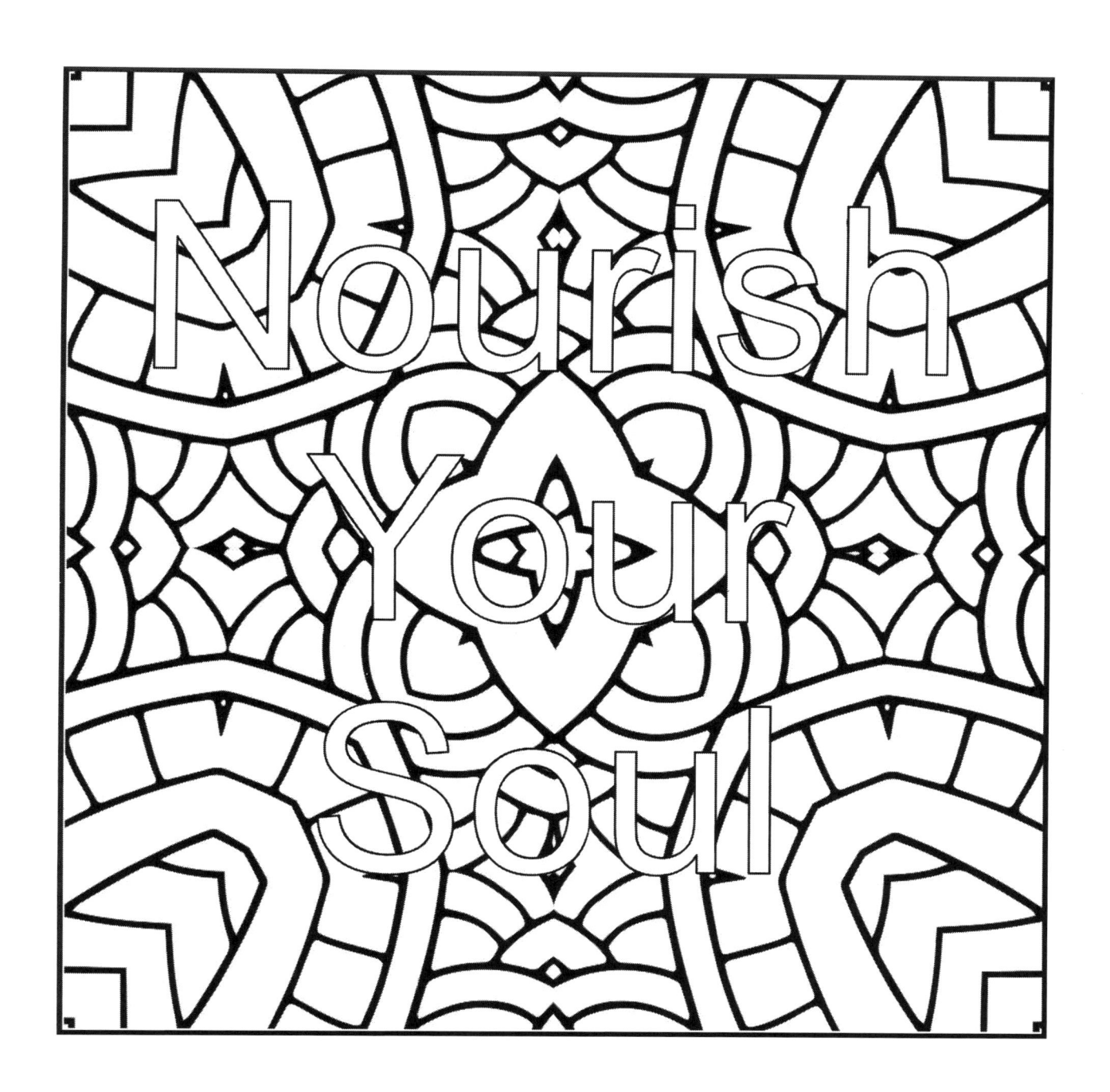

Persistence

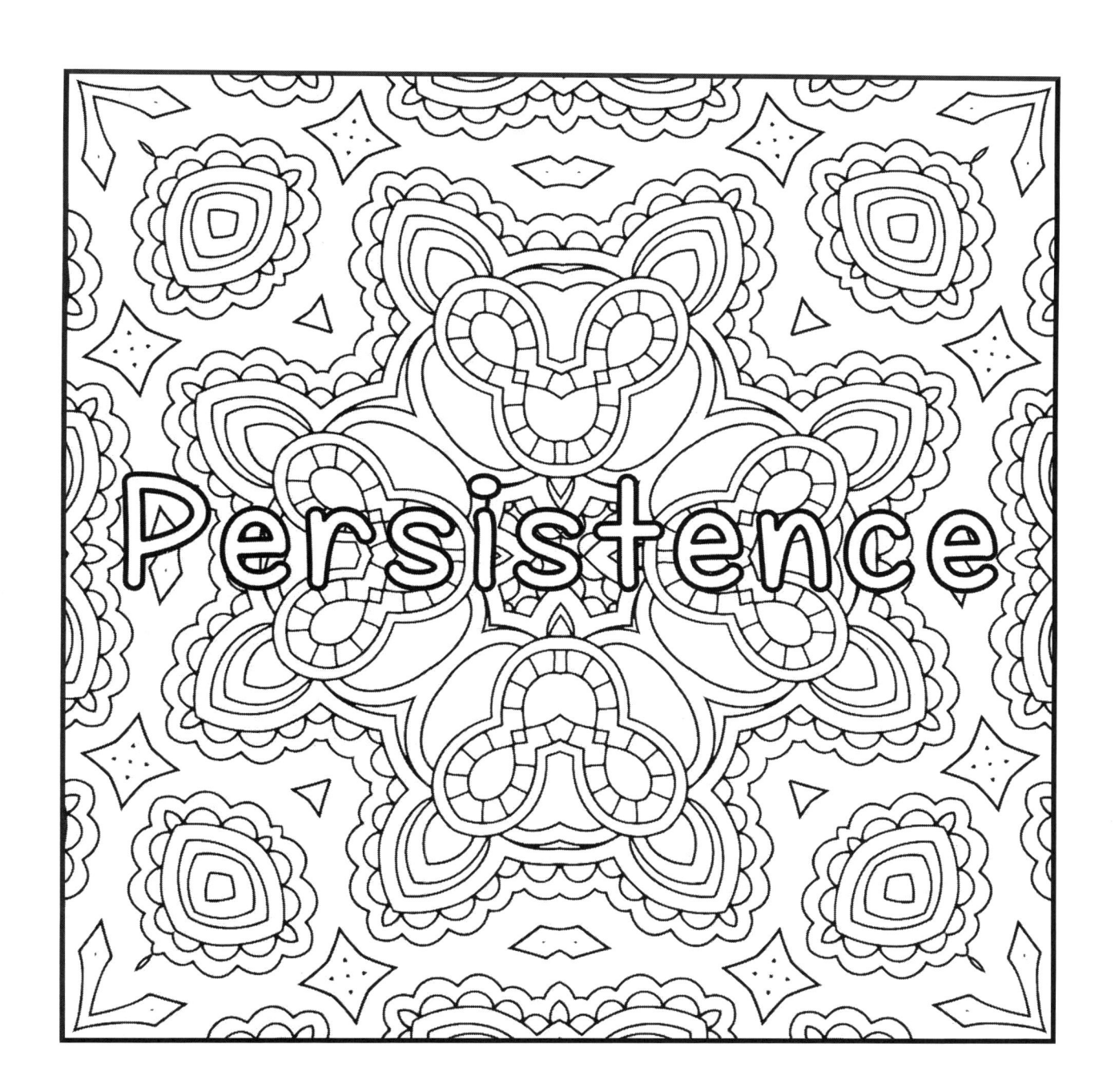

Keep Going

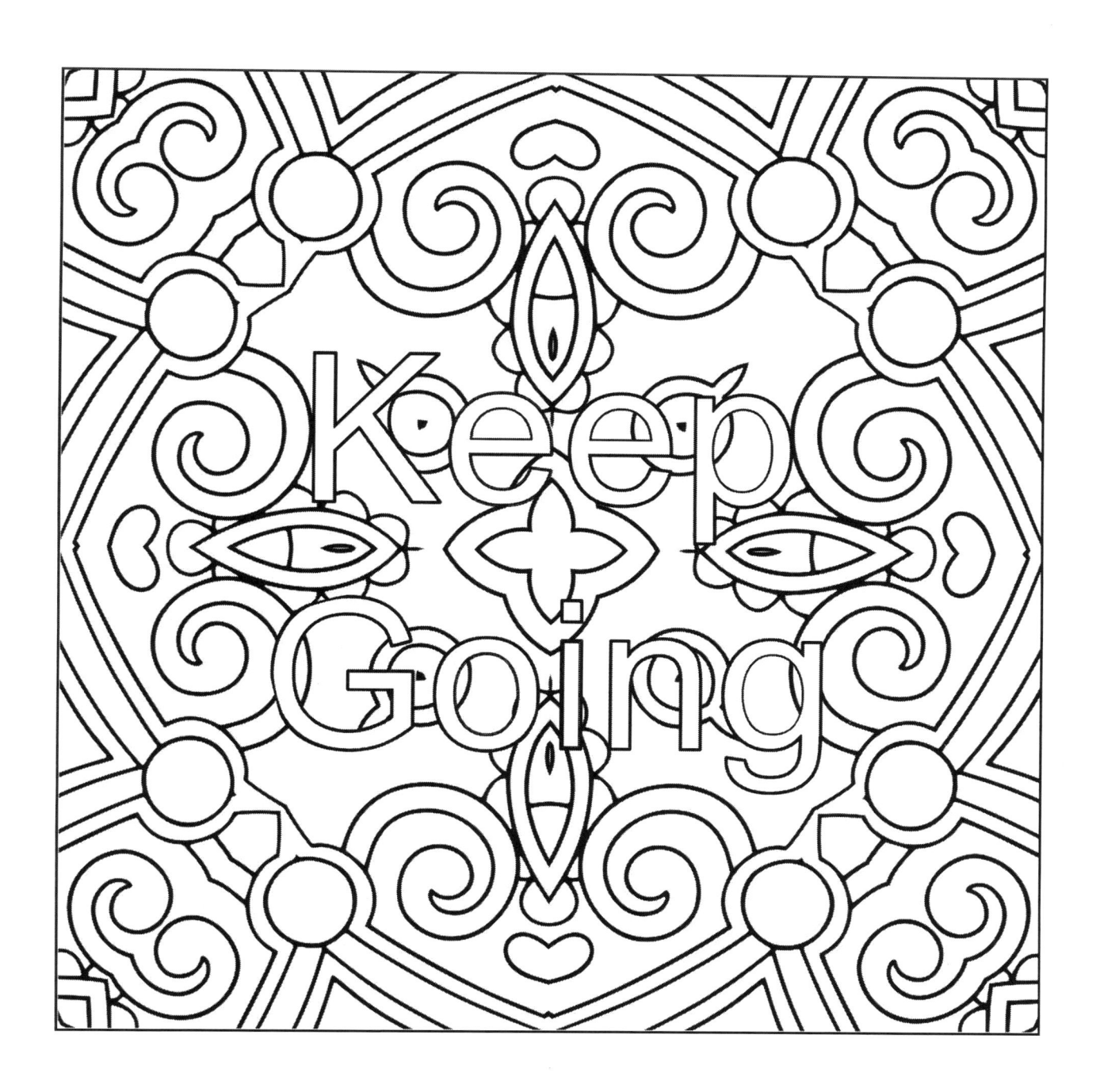

Be True to Yourself

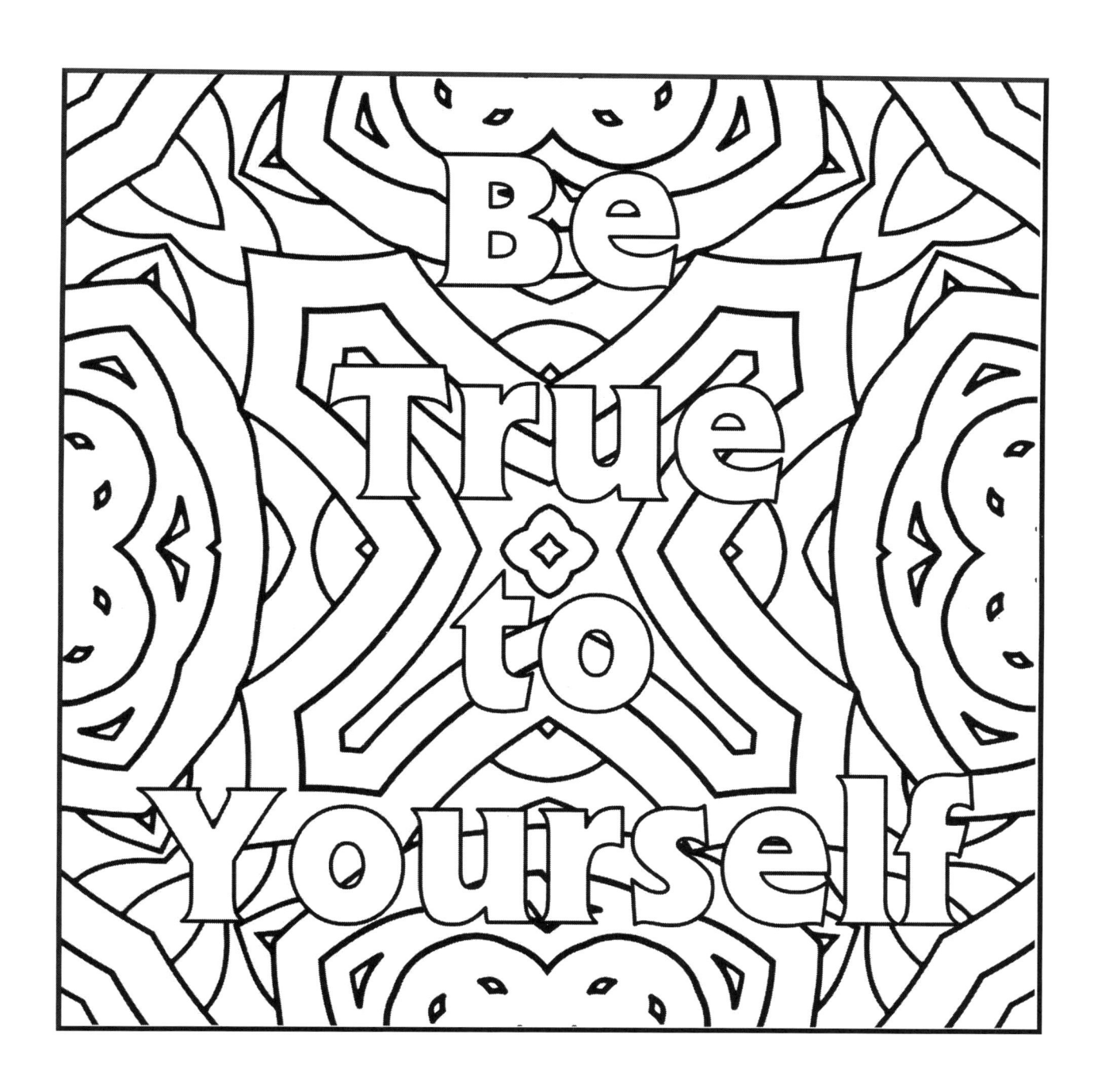

Did I Eat That?

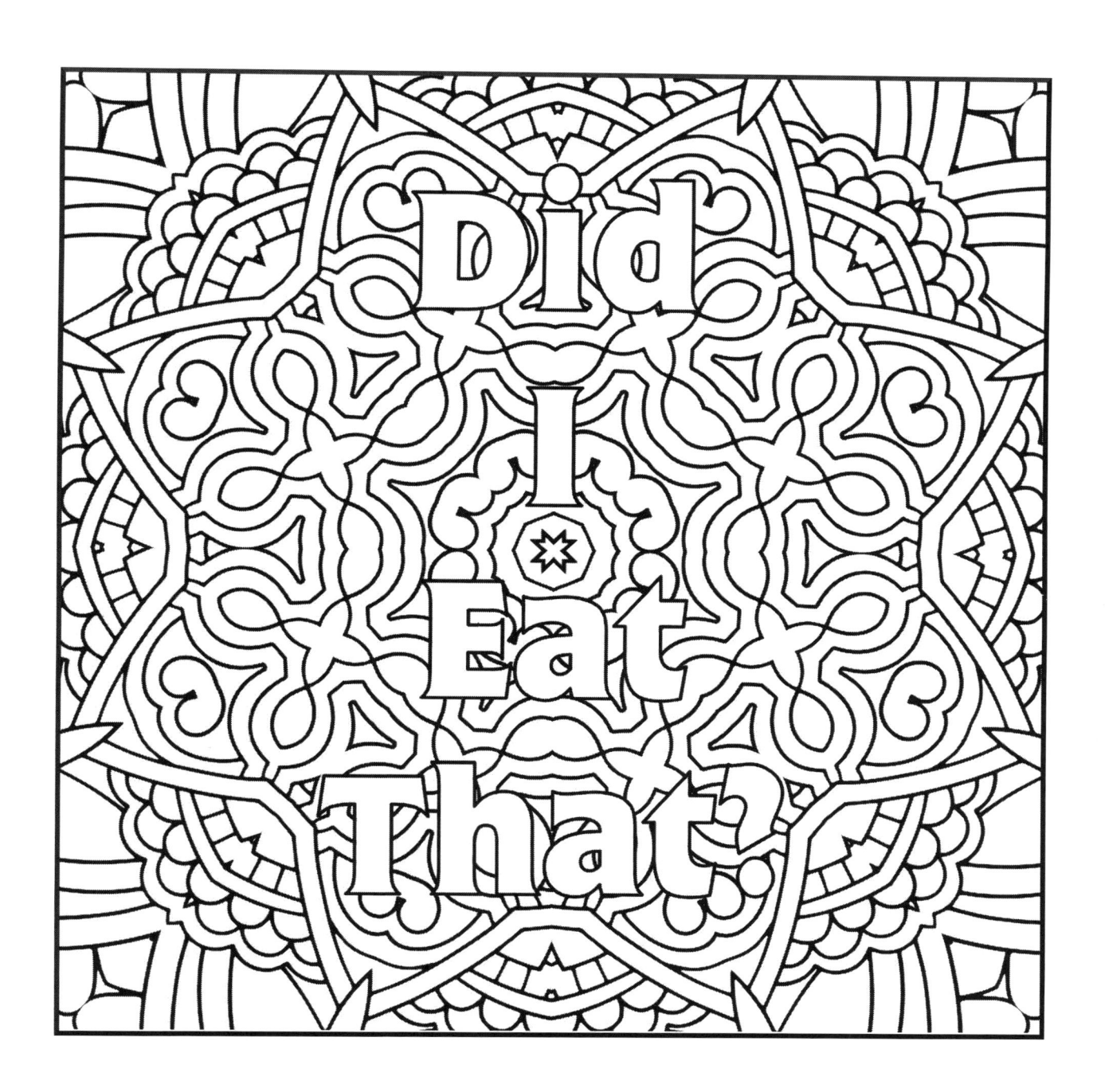

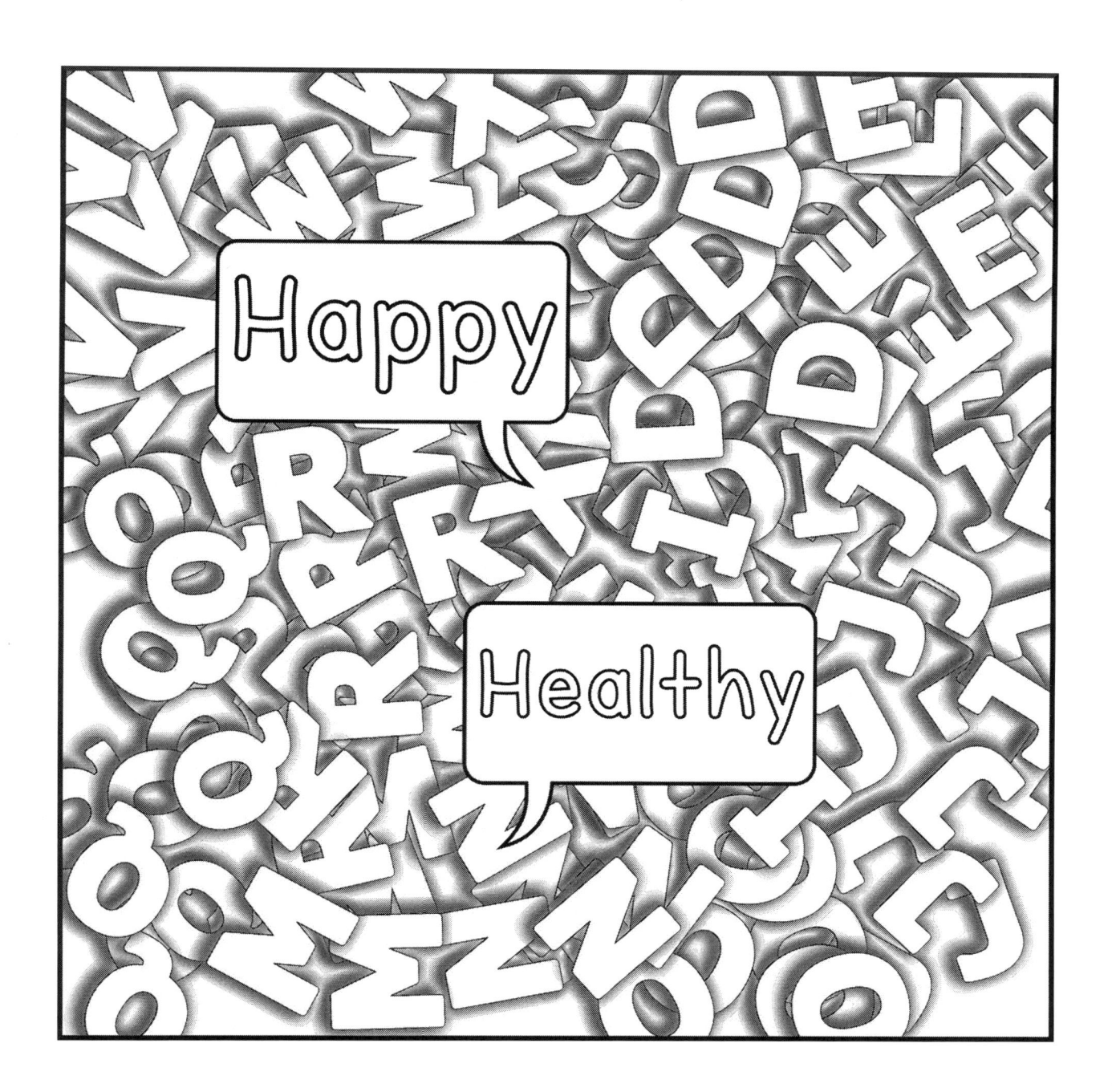

Mind Over Matter

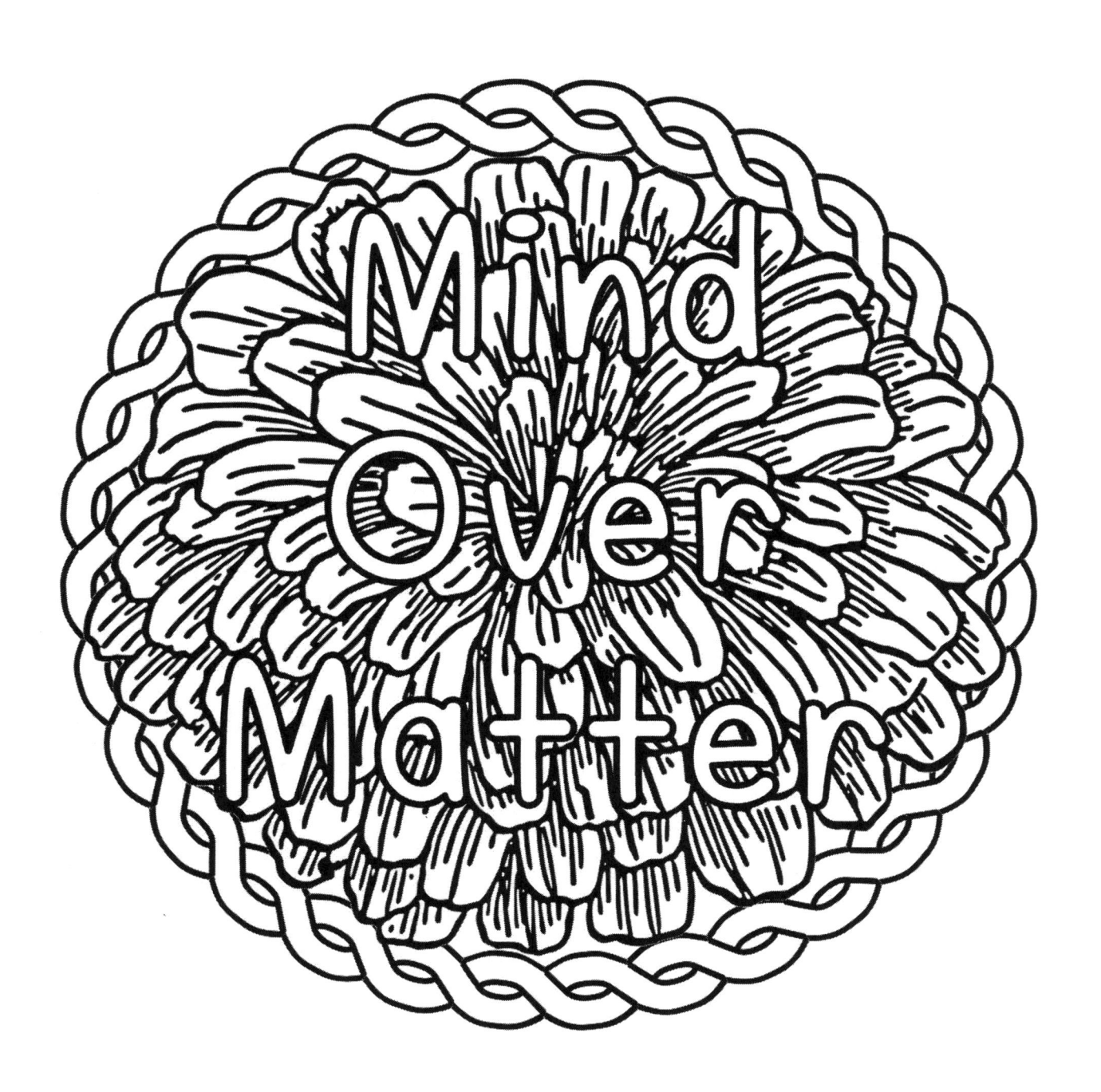

Staying the Course

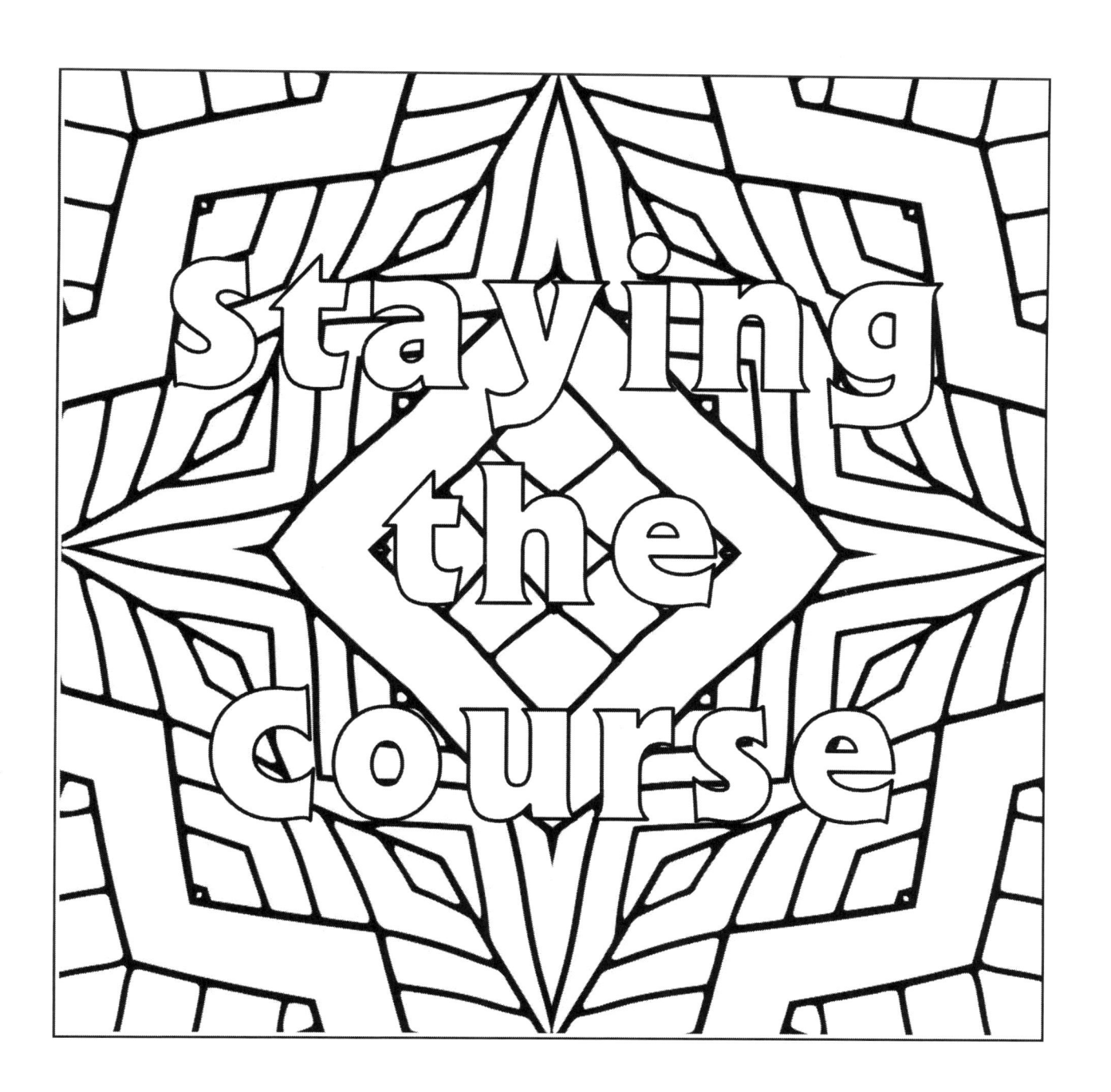

Moderation

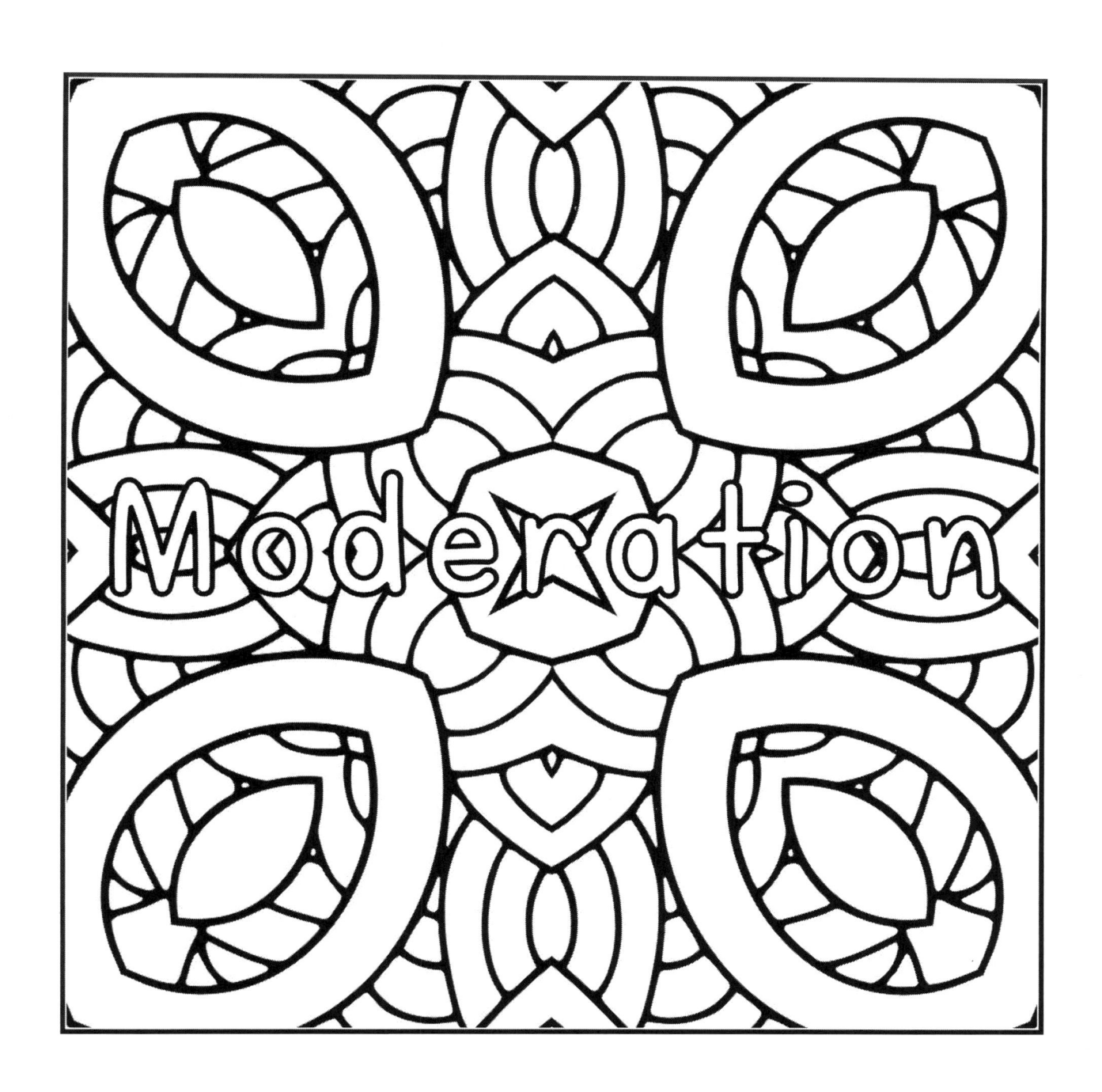

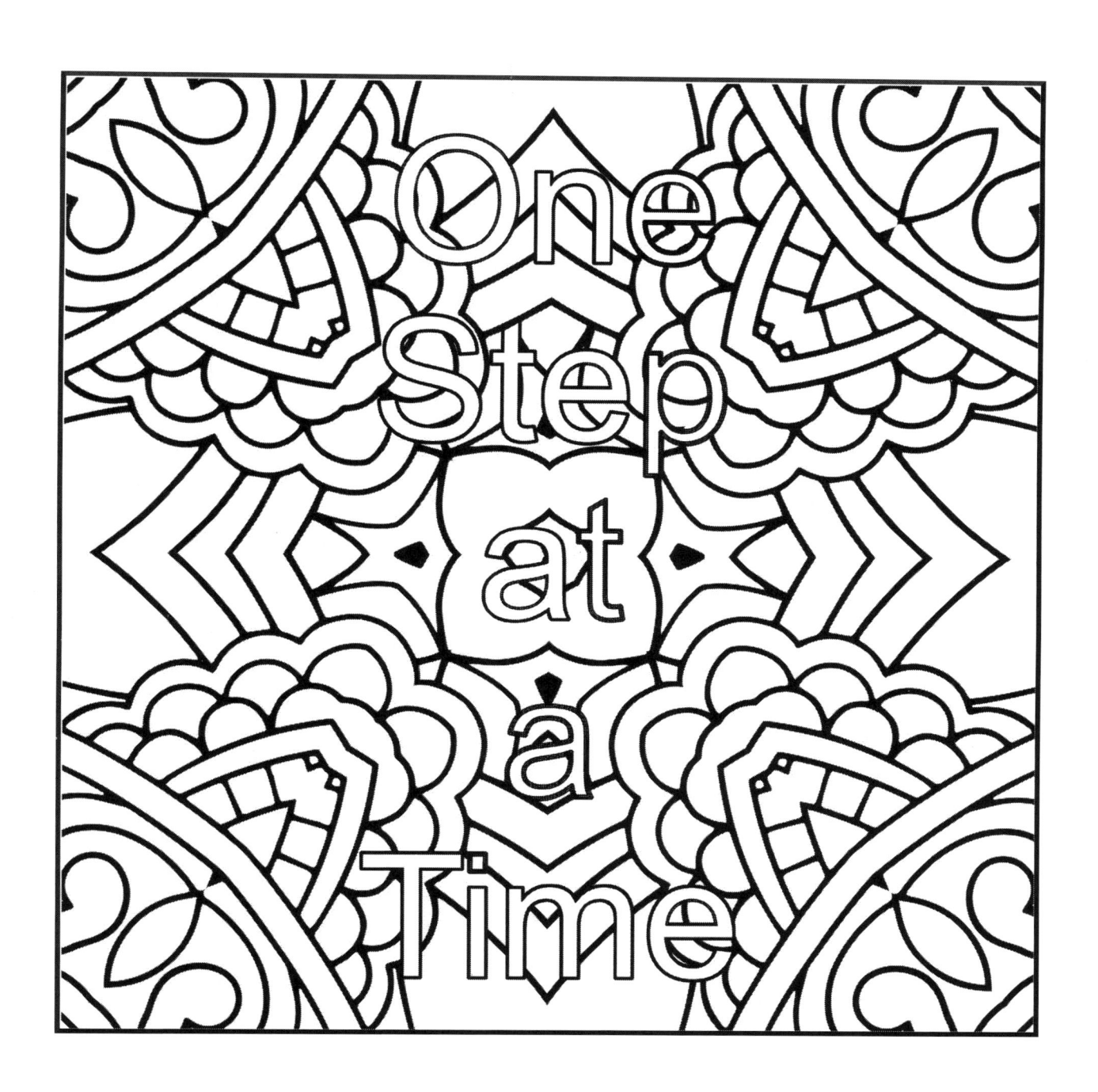

Exercise Body and Mind

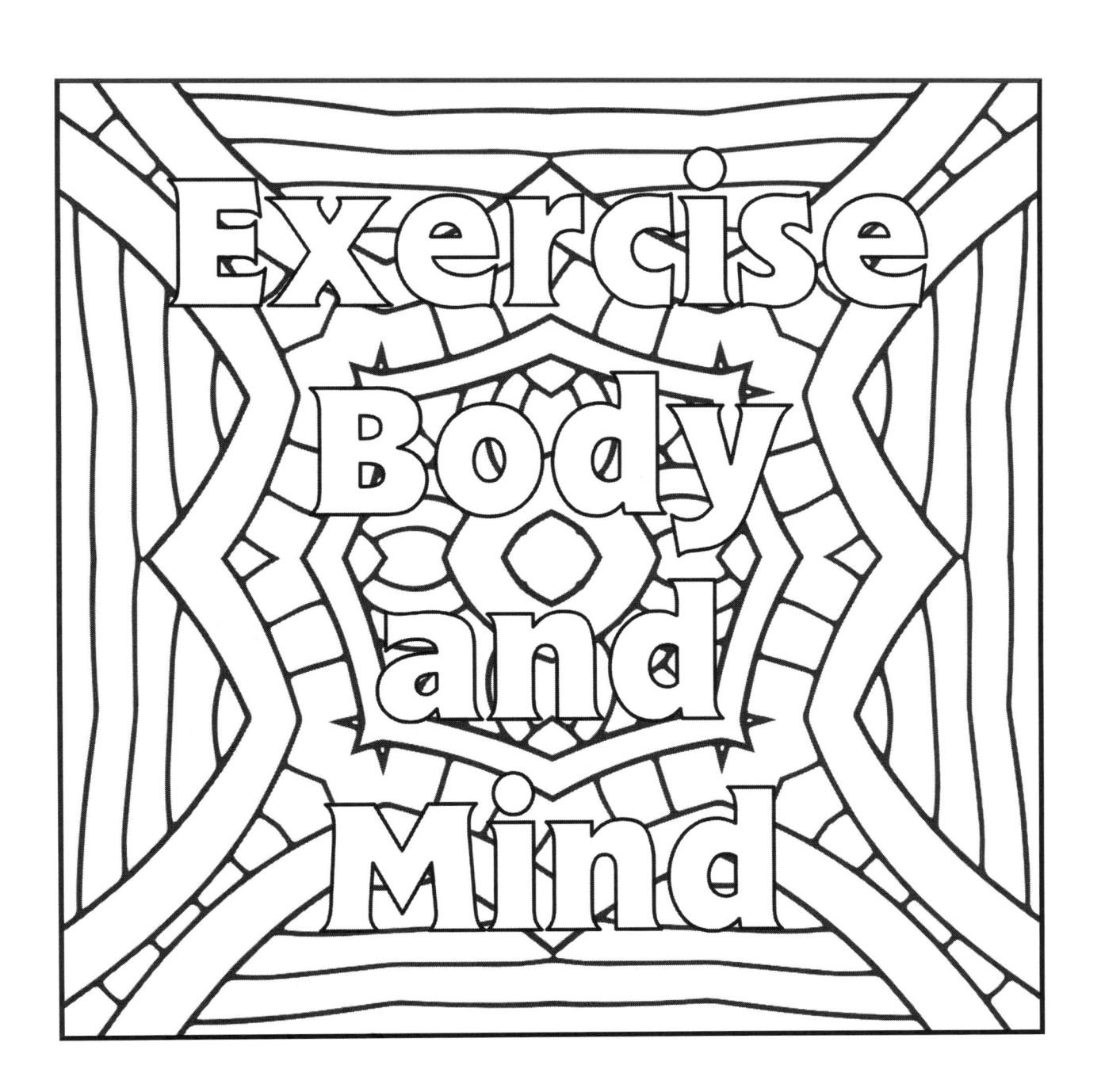

Healthy Goals

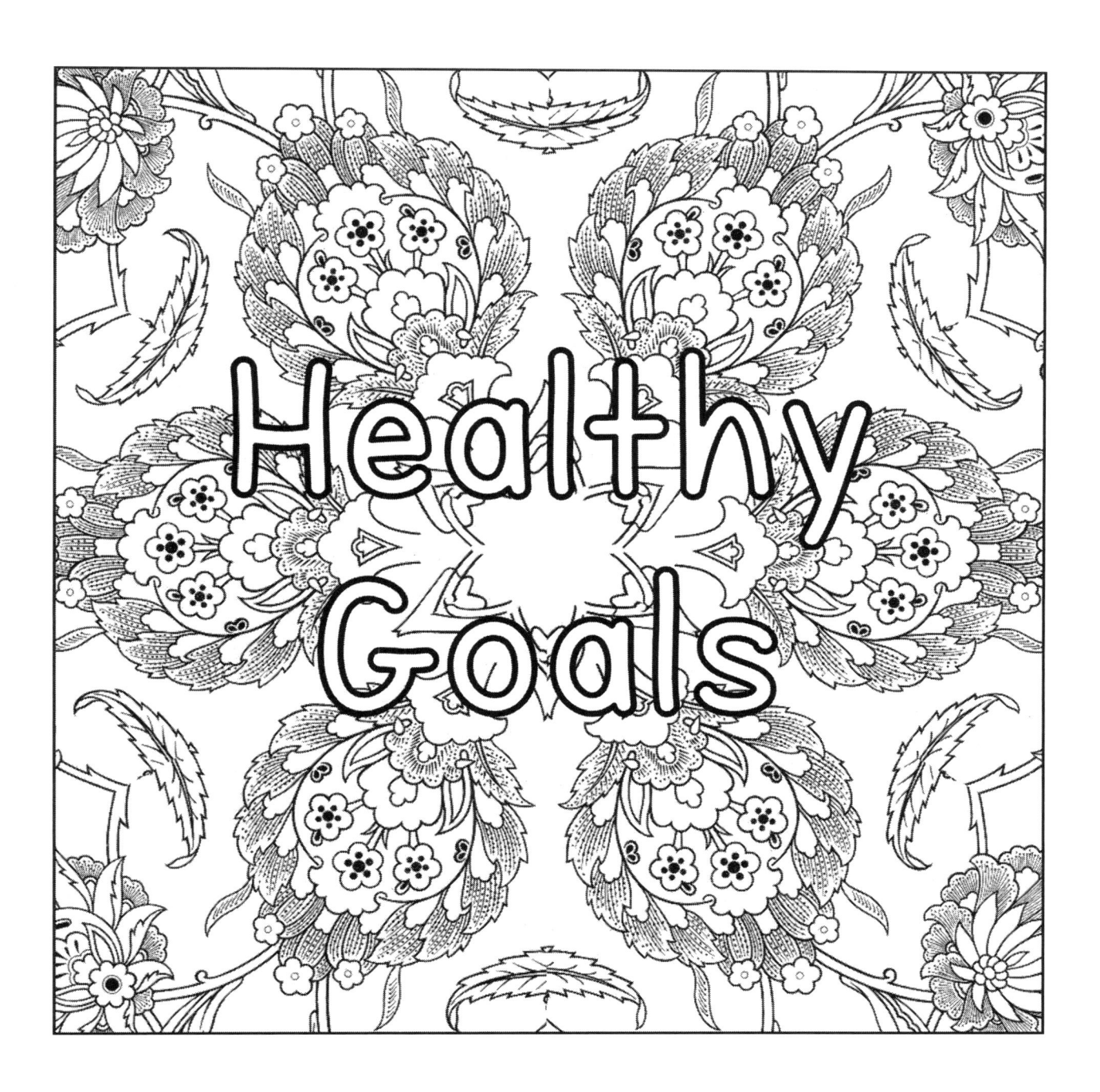

Love Yourself Today

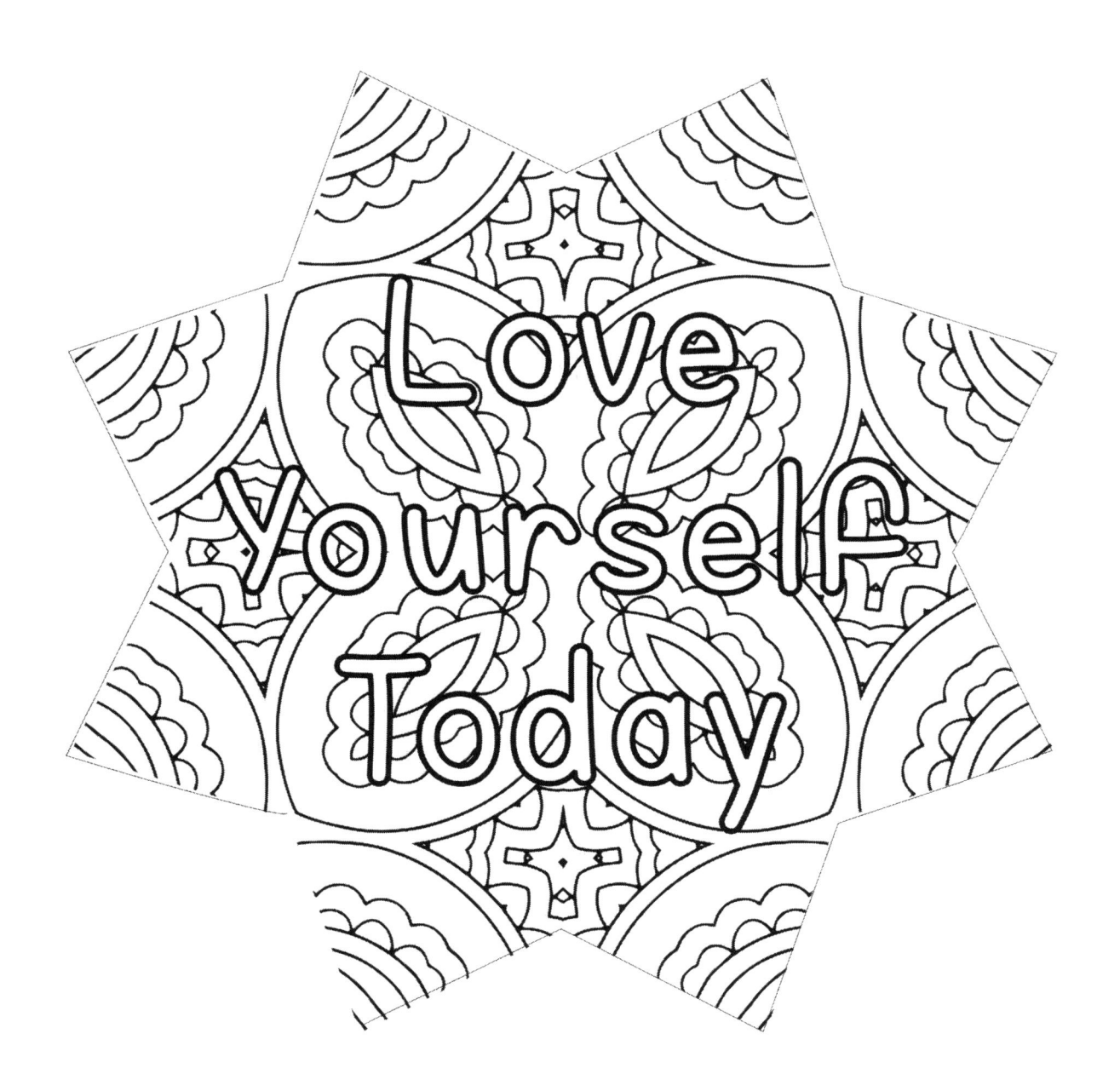

Strive and Win

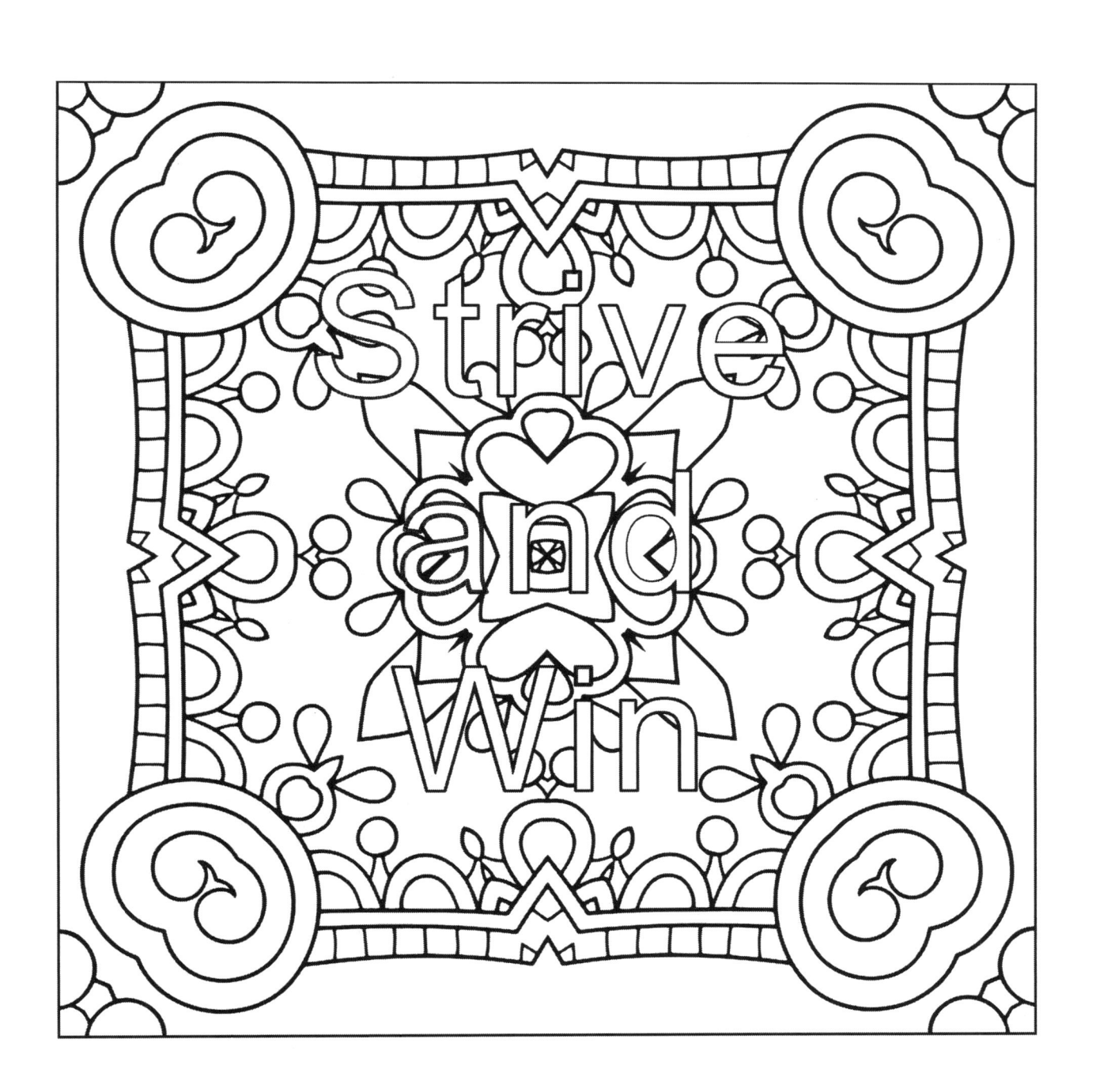

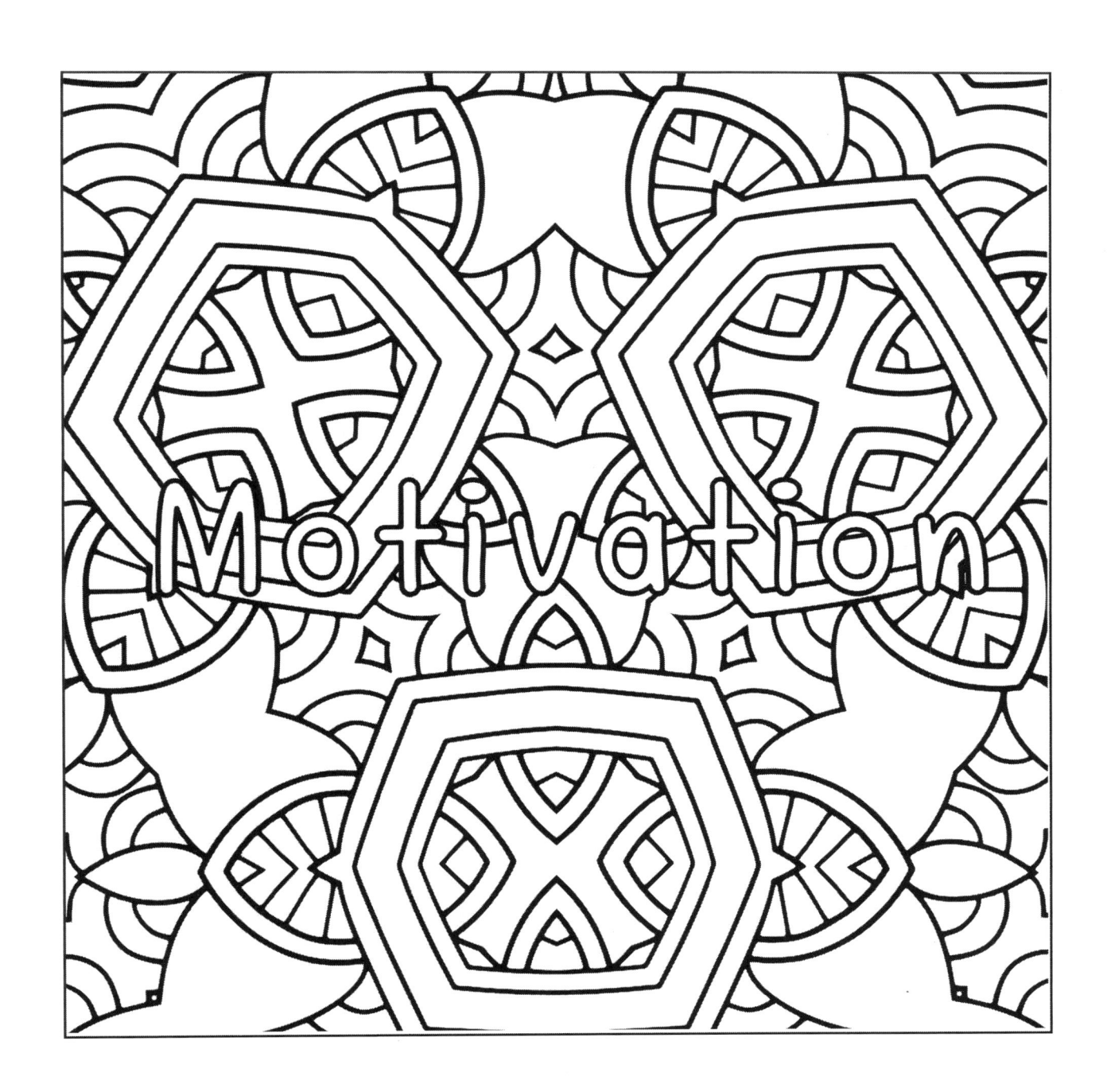

Motivation

Better Than Yesterday

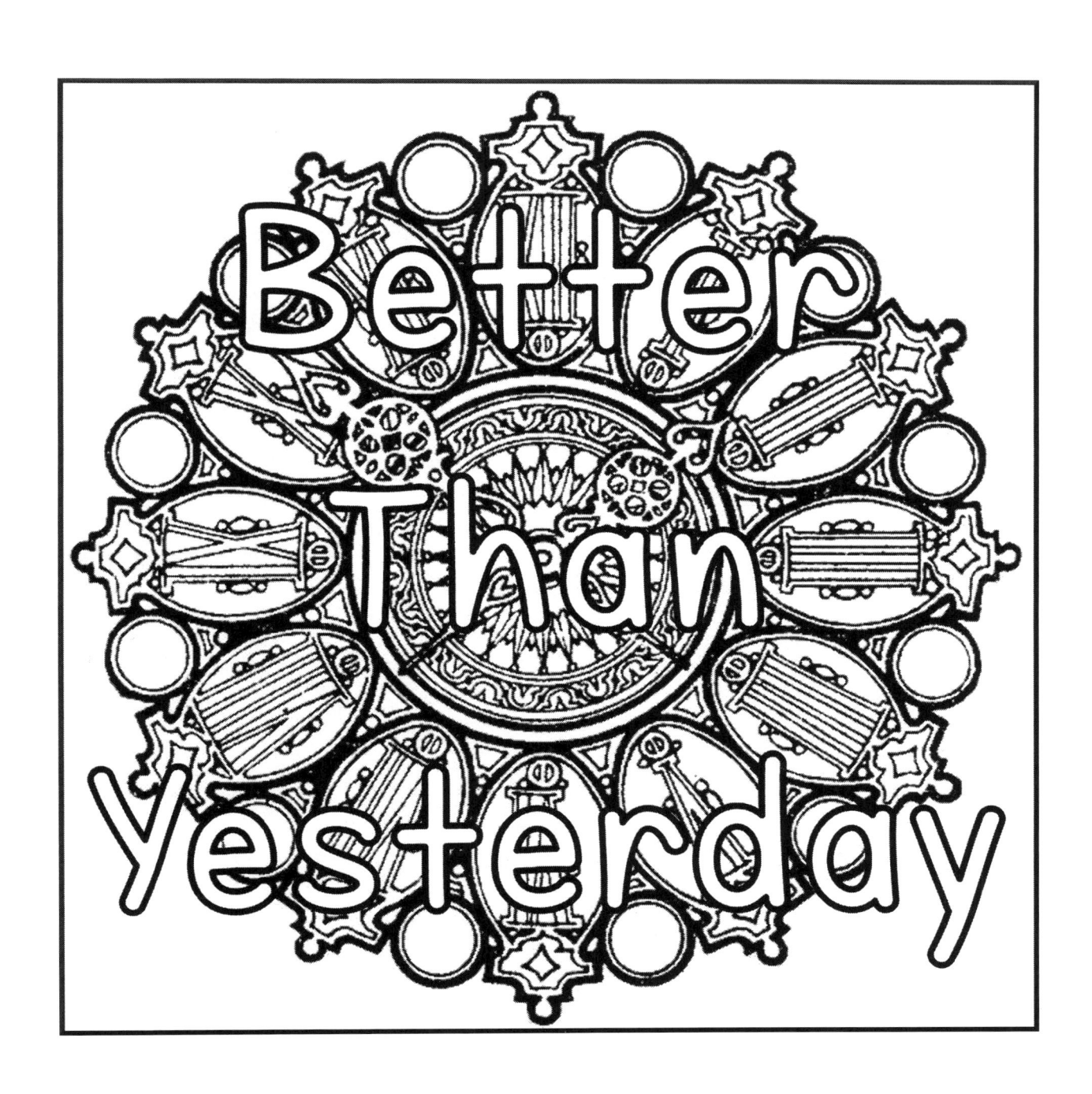

Doing Great

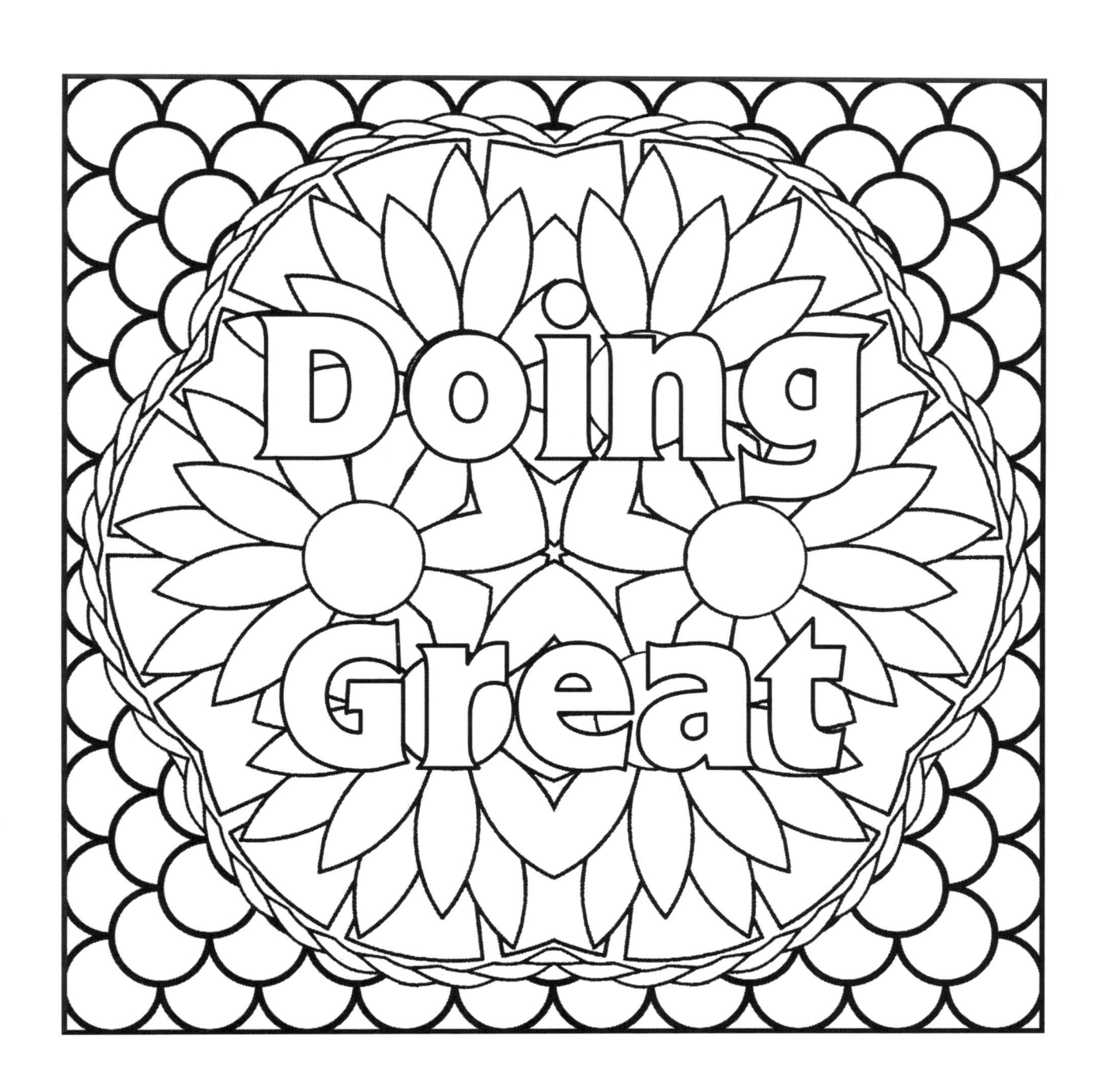

Mindful Eating

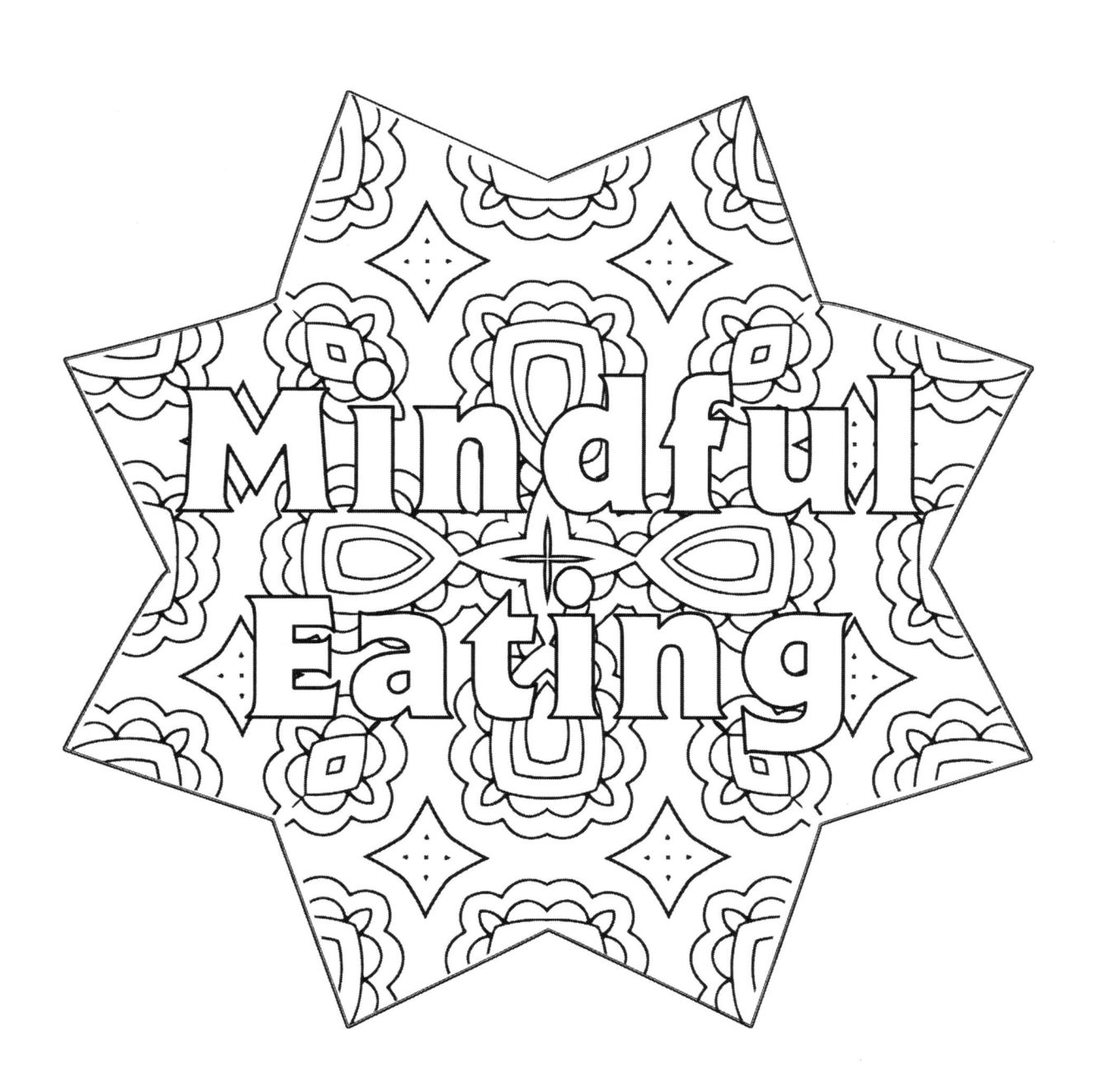

Feed Your Spirit

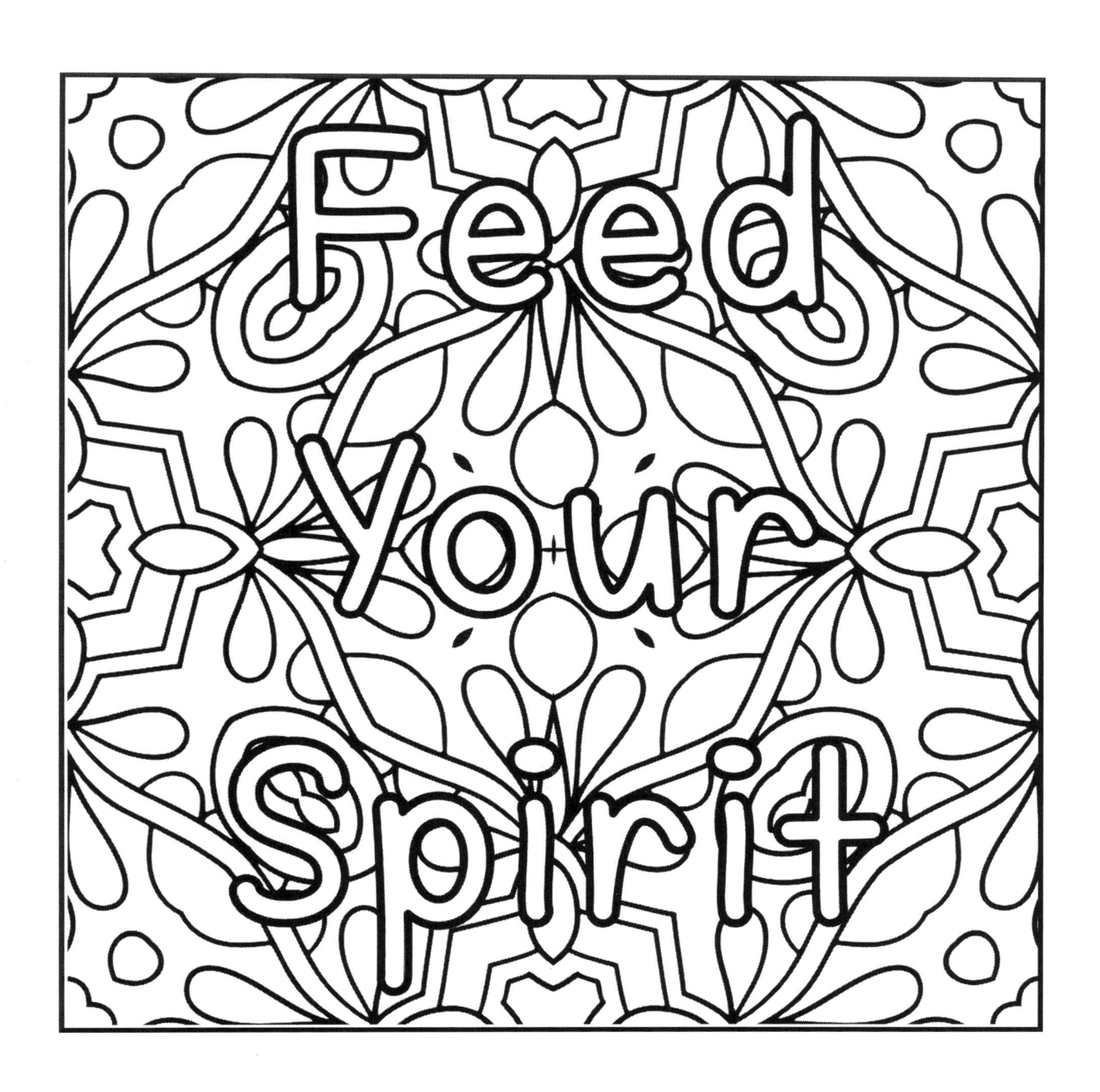

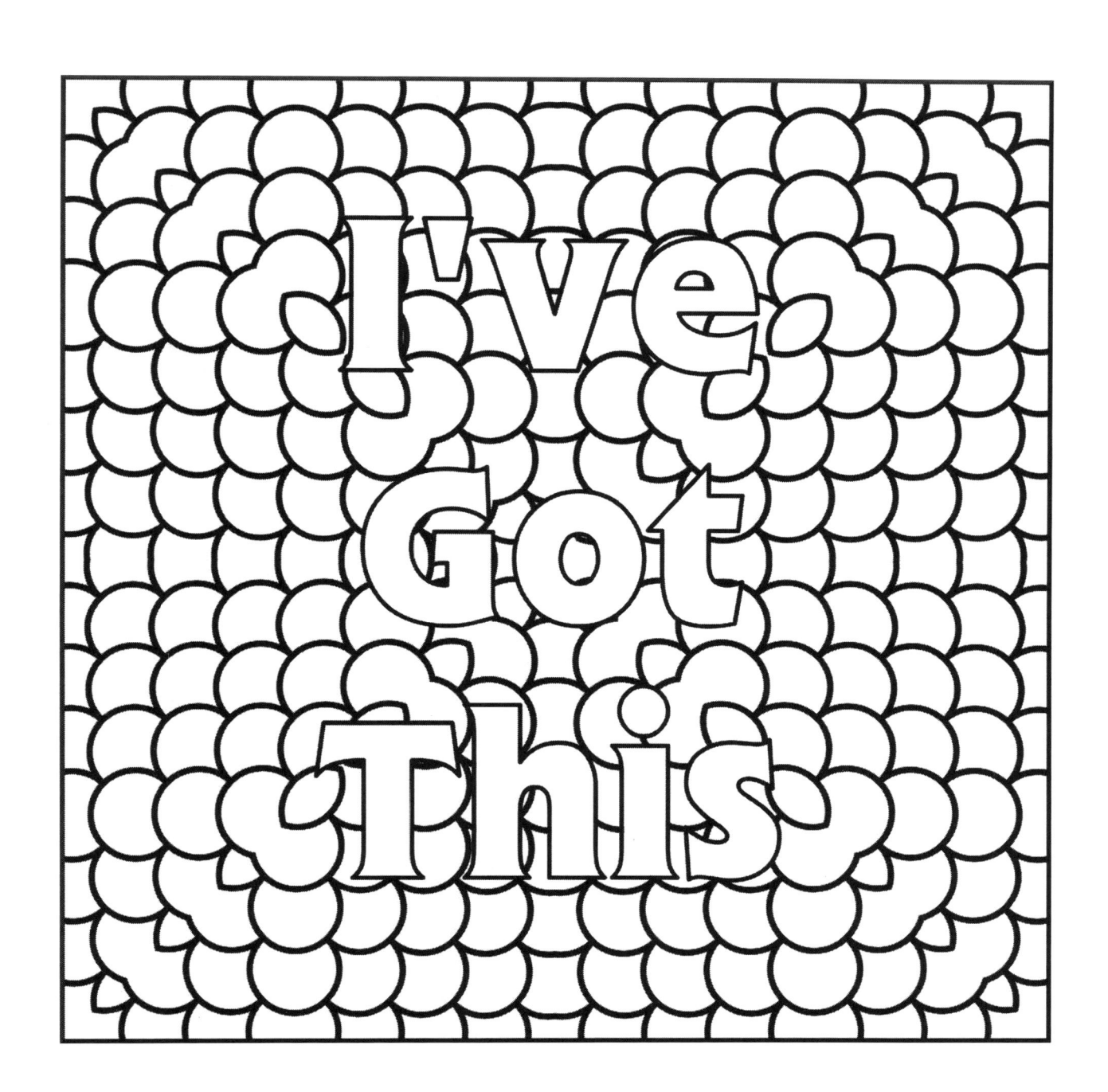

I've Got This

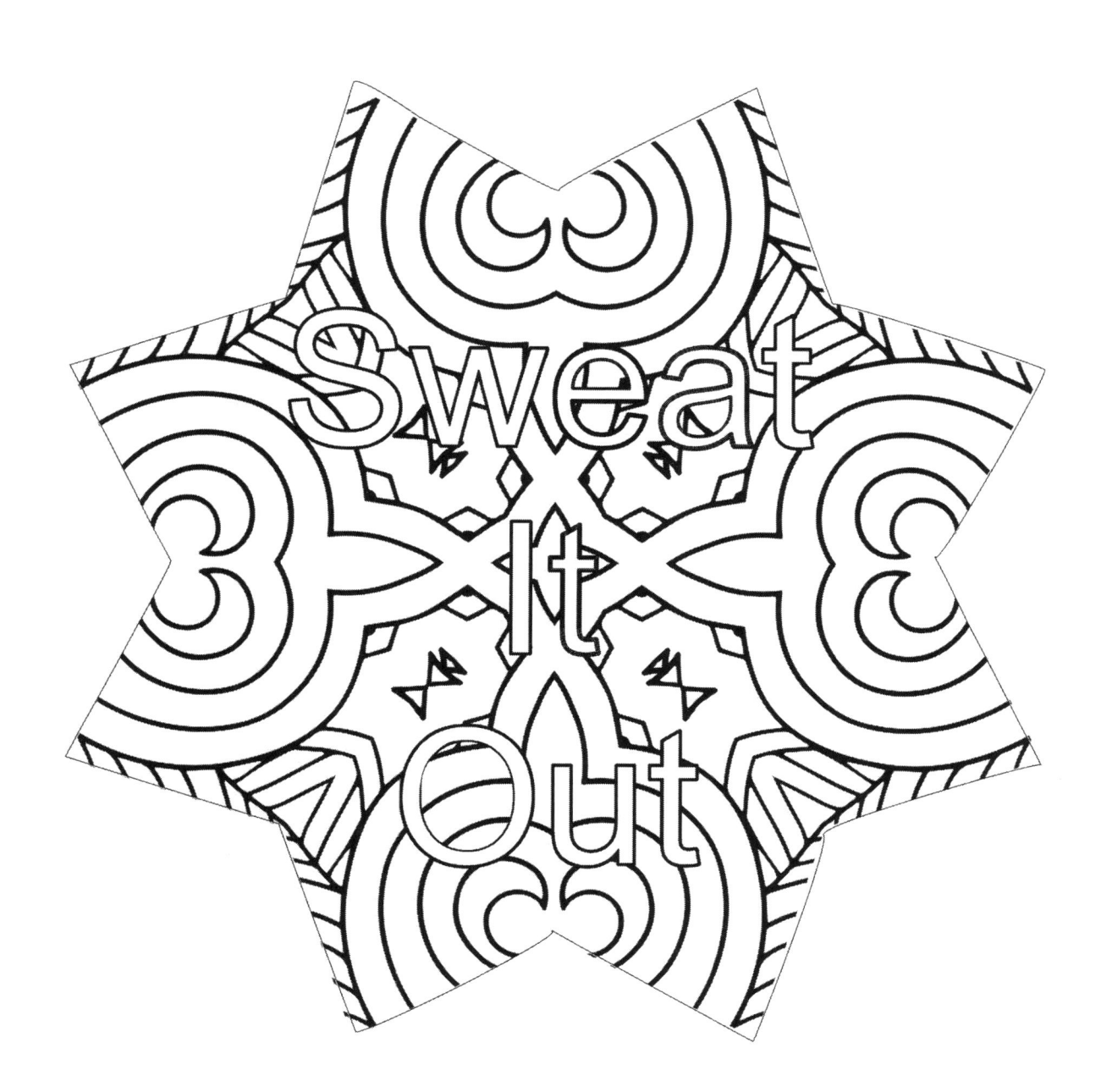

Water for Life

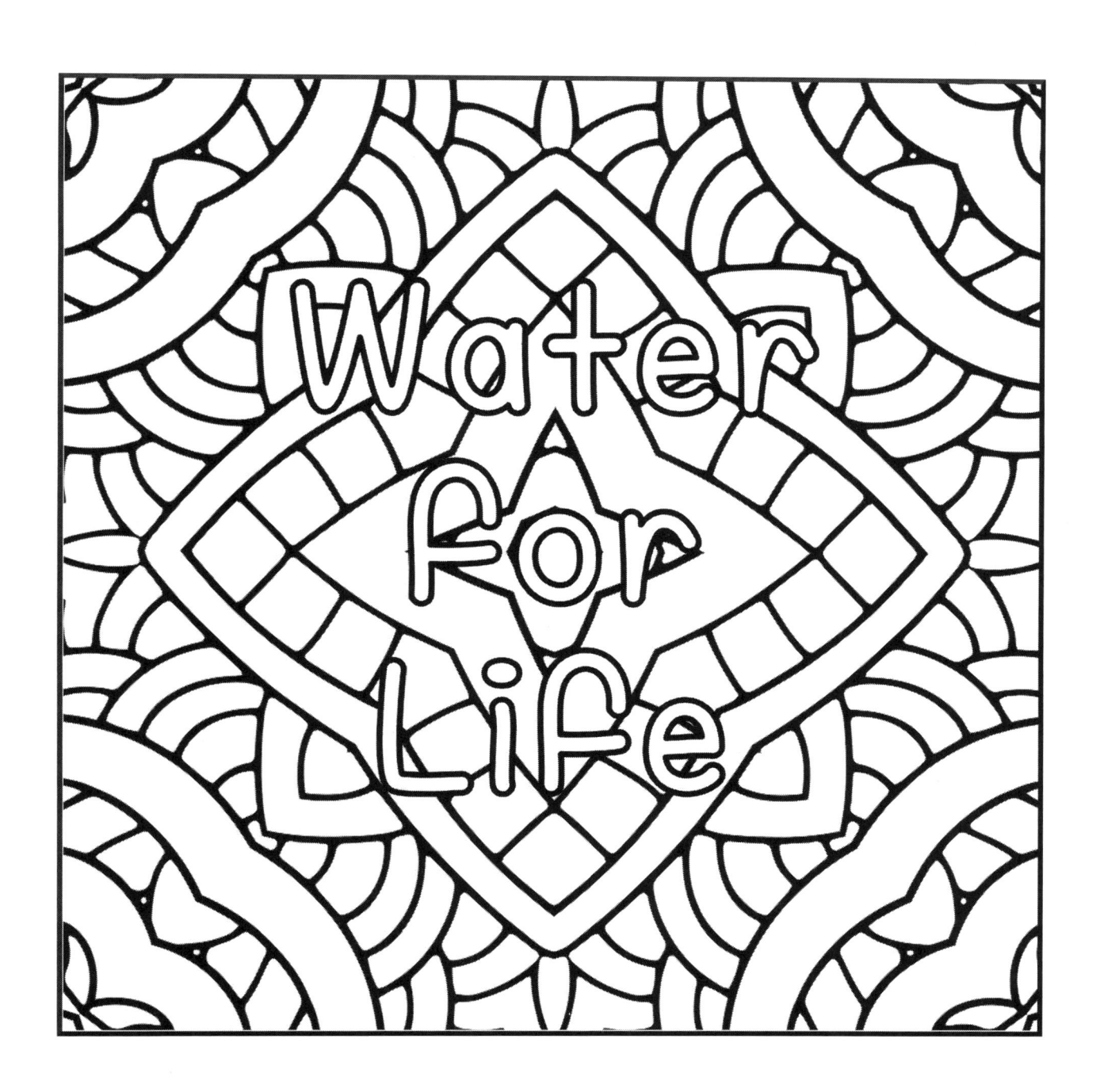

Eat Your Veggies

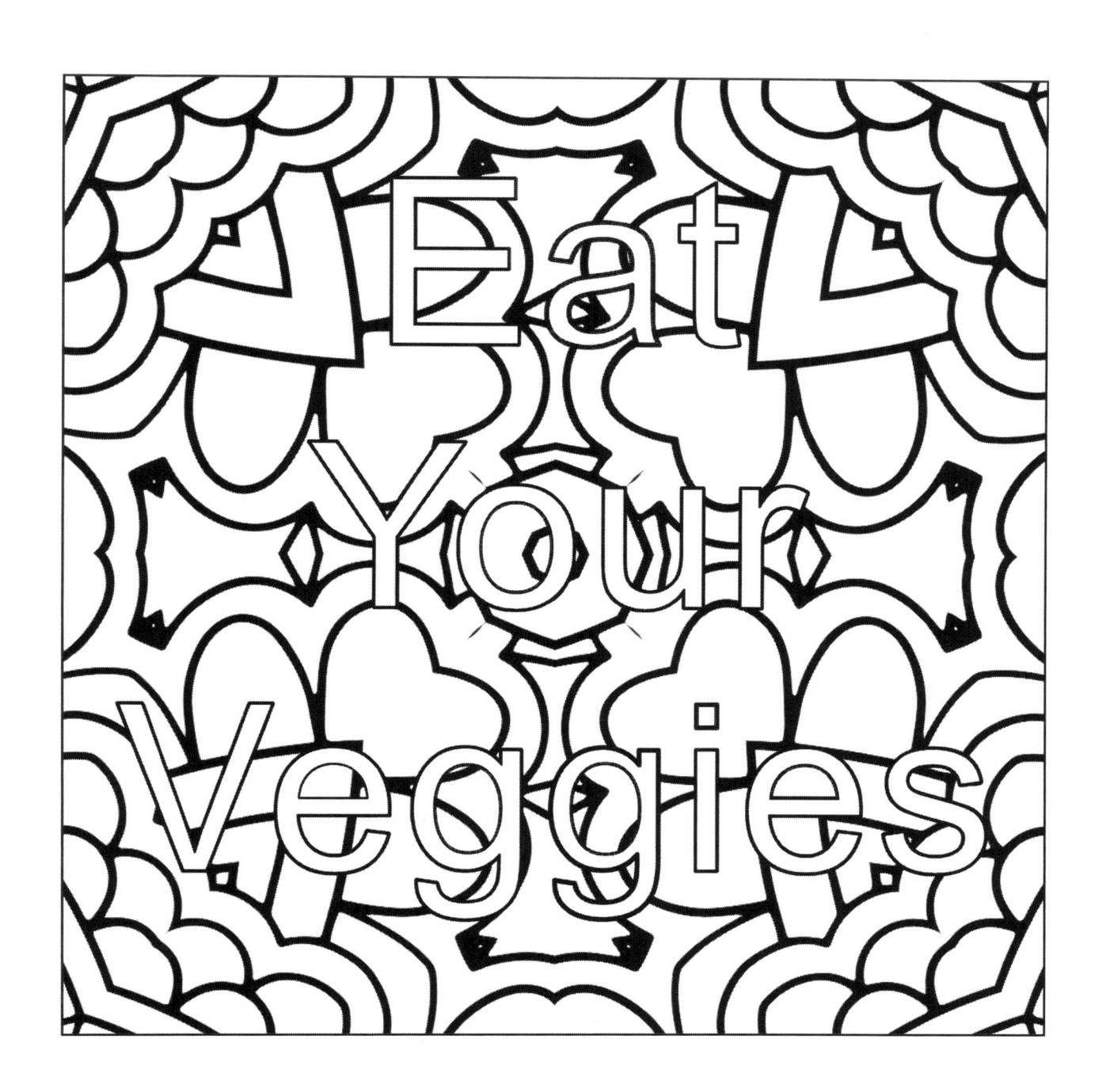

Fitness

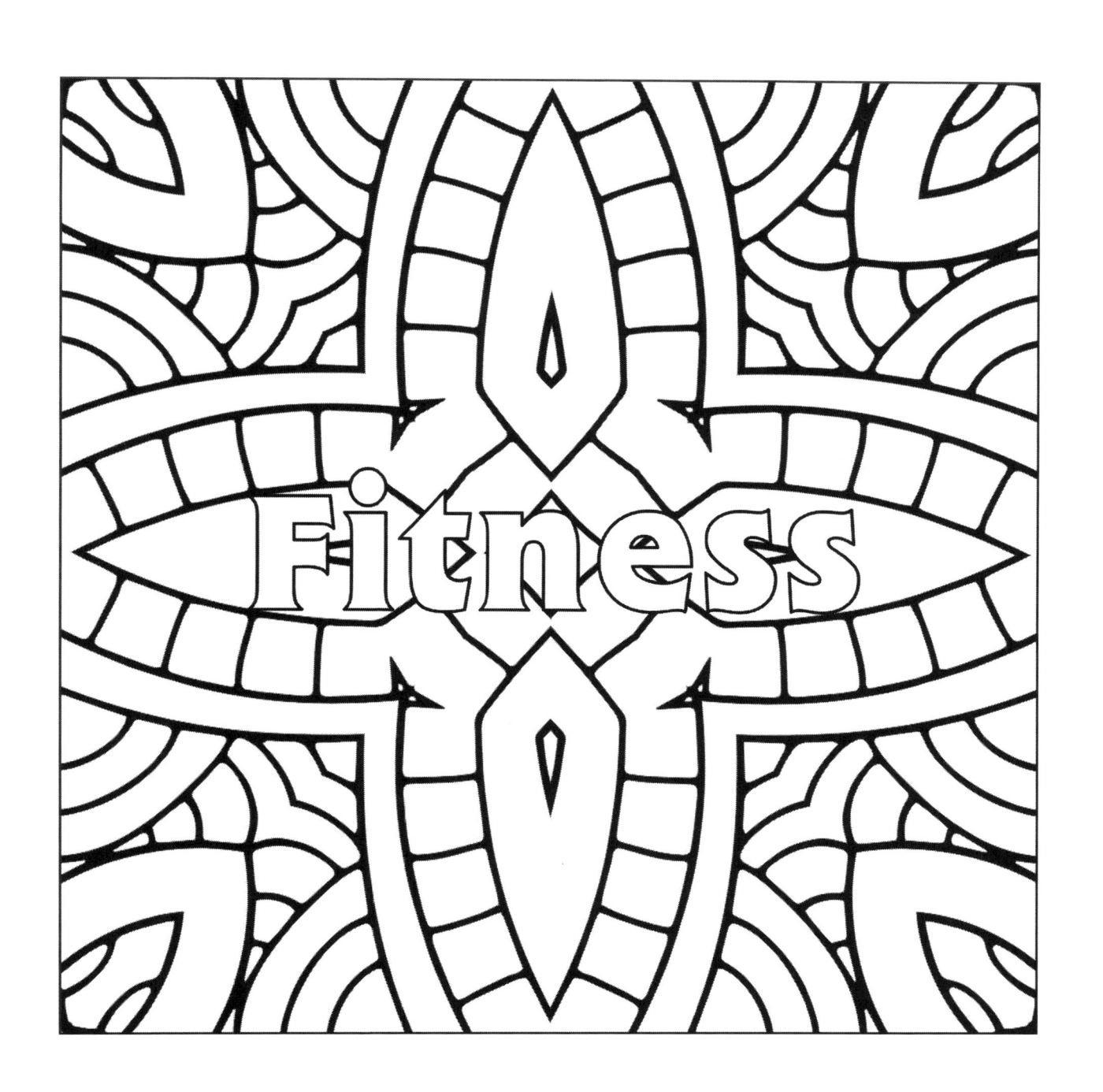

More Fit

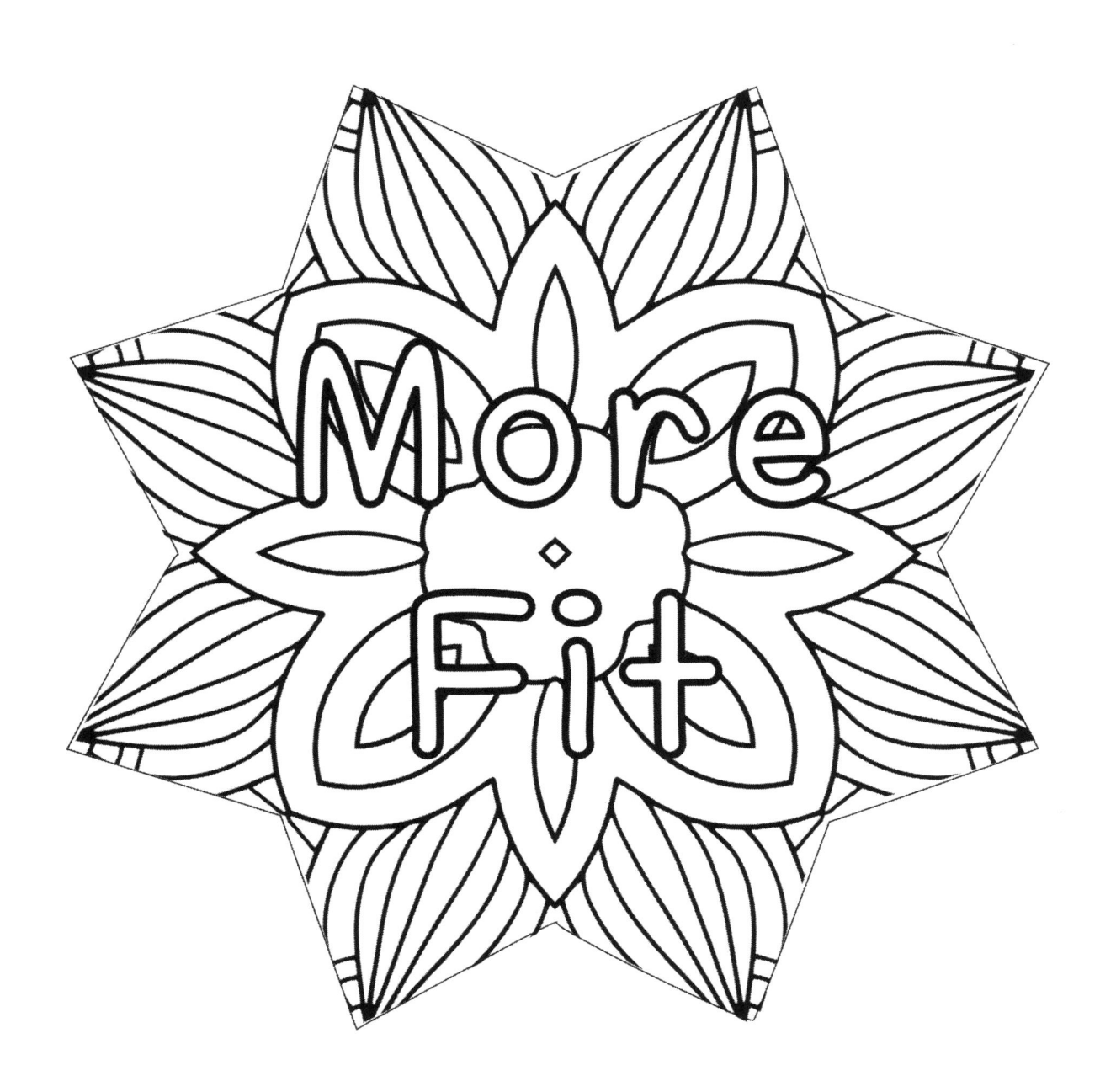